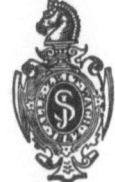

Recent Results in Cancer Research

Fortschritte der Krebsforschung

Progrès dans les recherches sur le cancer

24

Edited by

Springer-Verlag Berlin · Heidelberg · New York 1970

Recent Results in Cancer Research

Fortschritte der Krebsforschung

Progrès dans les recherches sur le cancer

24

Edited by

V. G. Allfrey, New York · M. Allgöwer, Basel · K. H. Bauer, Heidelberg
I. Berenblum, Rehovoth · F. Bergel, London · J. Bernard, Paris · W. Bernhard,
Villejuif · N. N. Blokhin, Moskva · H. E. Bock, Tübingen · P. Bucalossi,
Milano · A. V. Chaklin, Moskva · M. Chorazy, Gliwice · G. J. Cunningham,
Richmond · W. Dameshek, Boston · M. Dargent, Lyon · G. Della Porta,
Milano · P. Denoix, Villejuif · R. Dulbecco, La Jolla · H. Eagle, New York ·
R. Eker, Oslo · P. Grabar, Paris · H. Hamperl, Bonn · R. J. C. Harris, London ·
E. Hecker, Heidelberg · R. Herbeuval, Nancy · J. Higginson, Lyon ·
W. C. Hueper, Fort Myers · H. Isliker, Lausanne · D. A. Karnofsky, New York ·
J. Kieler, København · G. Klein, Stockholm · H. Koprowski, Philadelphia ·
L. G. Koss, New York · G. Martz, Zürich · G. Mathé, Villejuif ·
O. Mühlbock, Amsterdam · W. Nakahara, Tokyo · V. R. Potter, Madison ·
A. B. Sabin, Charleston · L. Sachs, Rehovoth · E. A. Saxén, Helsinki ·
W. Szybalski, Madison · H. Tagnon, Bruxelles · R. M. Taylor, Toronto ·
A. Tissières, Genève · E. Uehlinger, Zürich · R. W. Wissler, Chicago ·
T. Yoshida, Tokyo

Editor in chief

P. Rentchnick, Geneva

Springer-Verlag Berlin · Heidelberg · New York 1970

Hormones and Human Breast Cancer

An Account of 15 Years Study

John Hayward

With 23 Figures

Springer-Verlag Berlin · Heidelberg · New York 1970

JOHN HAYWARD, F.R.C.S., Breast Clinic, Guy's Hospital
London S.E. 1/England

Sponsored by the Swiss League against Cancer

ISBN 978-3-642-87017-0   ISBN 978-3-642-87015-6 (eBook)
DOI 10.1007/978-3-642-87015-6

To Moo

———

We have failed in hundreds and thousands of cases; for years, for centuries past, we have failed to cure cancer as a local disease. Every excision of cancer followed by return is a failure; even the largest, the roughest, attempts to cure it as a local disease. If we can have any hope at all of curing cancer it must be in the study of it as a constitutional disease, for, so far as therapeutics yet have proceeded, nearly the whole power of therapeutics is that of constitutional remedies against constitutional diseases.   *Sir James Paget, 1874*

Foreword

Seventeen years ago Mr. HAYWARD came to work in the Breast Clinic at Guy's Hospital. At that time the influence of hormones on the progress of breast cancer was appreciated; the prescription of androgens and oestrogens in the treatment of the advanced case was well established, and the operations of adrenalectomy and hypophysectomy had recently been introduced. Nevertheless, the prevailing view of the nature of breast cancer was that it was a local malignancy which had to be eradicated before it spread too widely and only if that had occurred would the aid of hormones be enlisted. How these hormones worked was unknown, indeed, today, as Mr. HAYWARD points out, their mode of action is still unknown. What has happened, however, within the last seventeen years has been a change of emphasis in our views regarding the essential nature of this disease. Instead of breast cancer being considered primarily as a local fault spreading centrifugally, it is realised with increasing conviction that it is a generalised disease with local manifestations and that one of the principal, if not the principal, aberration from normality lies in the endocrine environment.

That this philosophy is demanding increasing acceptance is due in a significant measure to Mr. HAYWARD's own investigations. In this work he has had the devoted assistance of BRIDGET WOLFF of the Breast Clinic at Guy's Hospital and the expert collaboration of Dr. R. D. BULBROOK of the Imperial Cancer Research Fund. This book represents the distillation of seventeen years close study of the relevant world literature and the information derived from access to the two thousand seven hundred patients with cancer of the breast who have passed through the Clinic during this period.

In a colloquial sense this book may be described as "the last word" on the subject of hormones and human breast cancer; the last word that is to say on the present position of our knowledge of the subject in that all the relevant information as we know it is here ready to hand. In another sense, however, the exciting feature of this book, with its description of the many trials and investigations at present being undertaken, particularly perhaps the description of the unique investigation being prosecuted on the island of Guernsey by the author himself, is that it is "an interim report". Here is the unfolding of a story of which we may at present be reading only the opening chapter; what the final message will be no-one can say. Nevertheless, the road which is now being followed by the author and by those many research workers throughout the world engaged in similar enquiries is, perhaps for the first time, well signposted. On this signpost are written the instructions for strict scientific enquiry, as opposed to those directing the traveller down the beguiling pathways of clinical impression and uncontrolled observation. We can but encourage those workers who accept the far sterner task of struggling with painfully slow steps up the slopes of real progress towards the summit of truth.

Mr. HAYWARD is to be congratulated on writing a book which is informed with this spirit and which deserves to become a guide and friend to all those who struggle to unravel the complexities of a disease which causes so much misery and destruction.

London, 19th December 1969   HEDLEY ATKINS

Preface

This book outlines what is known about the hormonal aspects of human breast cancer and how this knowledge has developed since the beginning of the century. Within this framework is given a detailed account of the results of fifteen years collaborative work undertaken in London by the Breast Unit at Guy's Hospital and the Section of Clinical Chemistry at the Imperial Cancer Research Fund. Rather than attempt to discuss the many thousands of relevant papers in the world literature, comparatively few key examples have been chosen to indicate the trend of current thinking. Where complete reviews are available, these have been mentioned in the appropriate section.

In essence, this book is simply intended for those who are interested in breast cancer, whether they be surgeons, physicians or research workers. I hope clinicians will find the material of some value in their practice and with this in mind I have given some conclusions and a summary at the end of each chapter. Those research workers who are not medically qualified may find information which will help to fill in some of the clinical background to their subject.

I owe a debt of thanks to many people. To successive secretaries who have had to decipher mountains of ill-written script; to Dr. J. W. MEAKIN who supplied much of the information used in the section on hypercalcaemia; to BRIDGET WOLFF who patiently corrected the bad English, and subsequently undertook the proofreading; and to Dr. R. D. BULBROOK who helpfully criticised the presentation, advised me on questions of fact and suggested the final format of the book.

May 1970   JOHN HAYWARD

Contents

Part II — The Hormonal Environment and Hormone Assays

Chapter 1

Historical Developments

An historical review of the endocrine factors involved in breast cancer gives little cause for complacency. After seventy years there is little knowledge of the basic principles involved and treatment by endocrine means is therefore empirical. The physician, in selecting the appropriate therapy for his patient, is still groping in the dark.

Yet an awareness of the advances that have been made over the years can be important, not only to the research worker so that he may gain an understanding of the background of the problem he is investigating, but also to the physician. It is the physician's responsibility to assess the suitability both of his patient for the treatment and of the treatment for his patient; he has to decide on the type of therapy, how often it should be applied and for how long; and eventually he has to appraise its succes or failure. And at all stages of this involvement he may be influenced by his knowledge of the progress of research and by the extent to which each advance has moulded his approach to the problem.

Animal Studies

It is not the purpose of this book to describe the great volume of work that has been carried out on hormones and breast tumours in animals. Indeed, the behaviour of tumours in animals may be quite unlike that of similar tumours in man. The hormones responsible for breast growth and development may be different and in fact few of the advances in the treatment of the human disease have resulted from animal studies. Nevertheless, the patterns of investigation have often run along similar lines and it is worthwhile considering the major developments that have occurred in the course of animal work—principally in mice.

As early as 1919, LEO LOEB, a worker of prodigious output, demonstrated that mice of a strain with a natural high incidence of breast cancer in non-breeders, had this incidence decreased when they were oophorectomised before three months of age. Subsequently, MURRAY (1928) showed the converse to be true; mammary tumours could be produced in castrated male mice when an ovary was grafted sub-cutaneously.

By 1932, both natural and synthetic steroids were becoming available and LACCASSAGNE published his classic paper on the development of breast cancer in male mice injected with "folliculin" benzoate (now known as oestrone benzoate) in oil. In 1935 ALEXANDER HADDOW, in a letter to Nature, described the retarding action of certain polycyclic hydrocarbons on the growth of the Jensen rat sarcoma. Many of these hydrocarbons were known carcinogens and it was noted that the greater their carcinogenic activity, the greater was their power to inhibit growth. Some

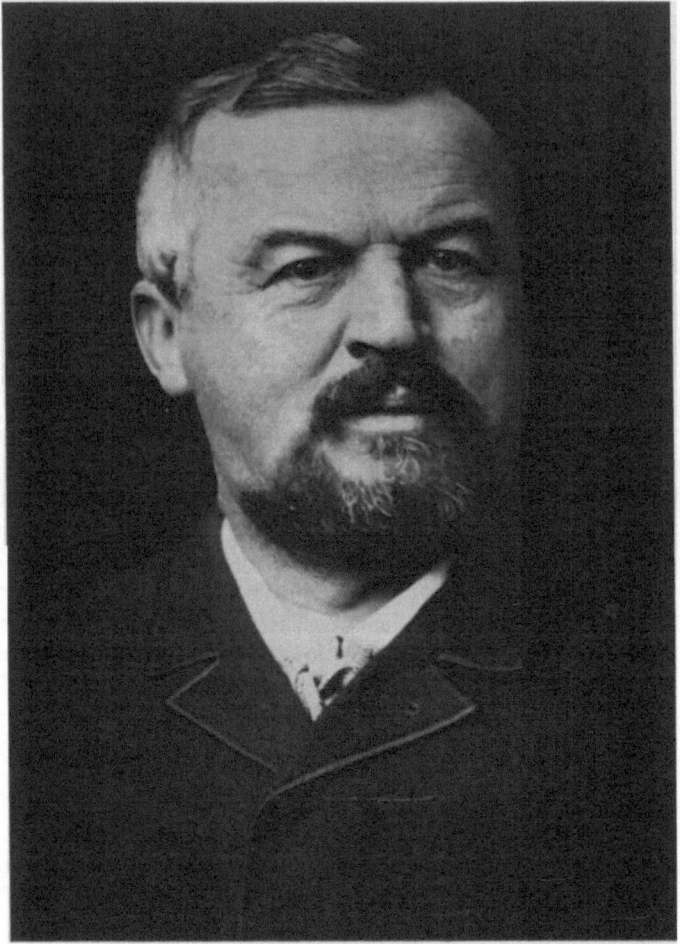

Plate 1. Prof. Dr. ALBERT SCHINZINGER. (Portrait supplied by Dr. ULRICH ROESEN,
St. Josefkrankenhaus, Freiburg)

of the carcinogens were also oestrogenic and hence attention was focussed on the
synthetic oestrogens which themselves behave as carcinogens under certain conditions
in animals. The results were encouraging and eventually a clinical trial was carried
out on the use of synthetic oestrogens in the treatment of human cancer.

In 1946 SHIMKIN and WYMAN further investigated the factors affecting the induction of breast cancer by oestrogens. They showed that the dose of oestrogens was
more important than the type of compound used. Male mice were implanted with
oestrogen pellets and it was calculated that the dose required to produce breast
tumours need not be greater than that secreted by the untreated female.

Following LOEB's (1919) finding that oophorectomy could be protective against
breast carcinoma in mice, KORTEWEG and THOMAS (1939) showed that hypophysectomy decreased the incidence of tumours in susceptible strains. More recently,
SHIMKIN and WYMAN (1945) have demonstrated that bilateral adrenalectomy with

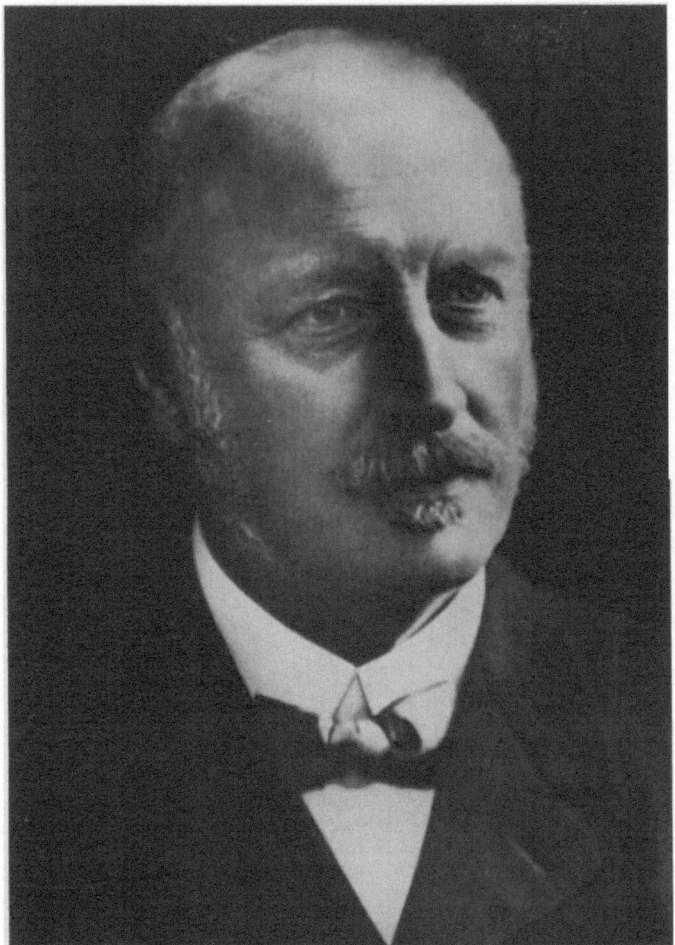

Plate 2. Sir GEORGE BEATSON. (Photograph supplied by Prof. A. P. H. FORREST and reproduced by courtesy of Dr. P. F. PEACOCK and Dr. J. PAUL, Beatson Memorial Hospital, Glasgow)

oophorectomy also decreases murine incidence of breast cancer. In 1949, FOULDS reported on a remarkable breast tumour which had a high spontaneous incidence in mice and was hormone responsive. If mice with this tumour became pregnant, the tumours in two-thirds of them grew during the pregnancy and regressed following parturition. In the other one-third of the animals, the tumour appeared to be unresponsive to hormones. It was also noted that the prescription of oestrogens did not affected the growth during the intermission phases.

In 1963, HUGGINS described the production of mammary carcinomas in Sprague-Dawley Rats following one feed of 9-10-dimethyl-1-2-benzanthracene. This extraordinary tumour can be completely "extinguished" by oophorectomy with adrenalectomy and stimulated to grow again by the administration of oestrogens. The Huggins tumour has proved to be one of the most useful animal systems for investigation.

1*

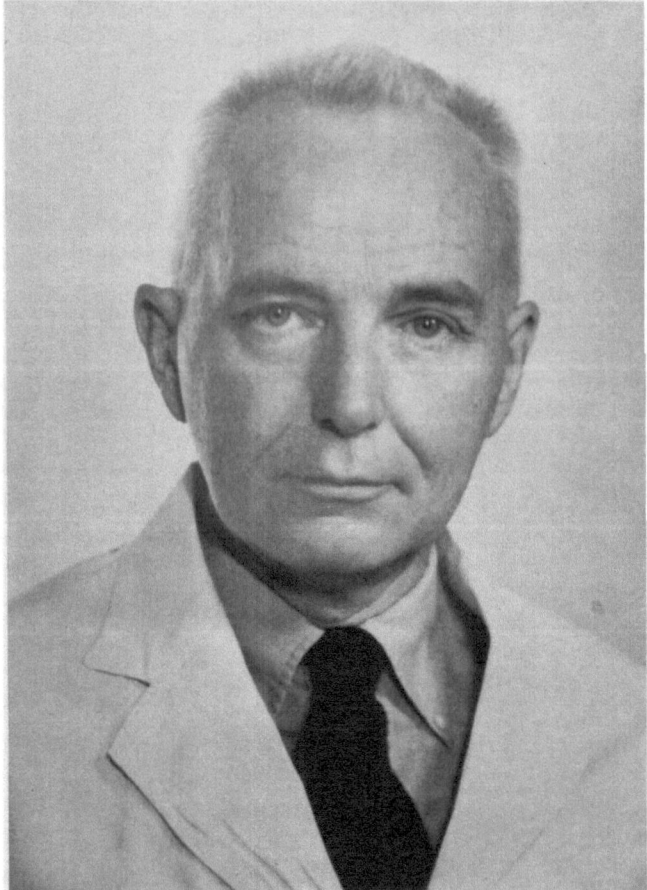

Plate 3. Dr. CHARLES HUGGINS

Human Studies

SCHINZINGER, a German physician, is credited with the first suggestion that there might be a relationship between the ovaries and human breast cancer. This suggestion was all the more extraordinary because at that time, the concept of hormones as chemical messengers was not formulated. In 1889, he suggested to the Eighteenth Congress of the German Surgical Association that removal of the ovaries in patients with breast cancer might cause the breast to atrophy, and result in the carcinoma becoming encapsulated in the contracting gland. So far as is known this was not put into practice and it remained for GEORGE BEATSON, a Surgeon at the Glasgow Cancer Hospital, to report on the first definitive removal of the ovaries as treatment for breast cancer. In 1896, BEATSON described to the Edinburgh Medico-Chirurgical Society, three patients with advanced breast cancer on two of whom he had per-formed bilateral salpingo-oophorectomy. Both patients had also received thyroid extract by mouth in the belief that this might act as a lymphatic stimulant. The

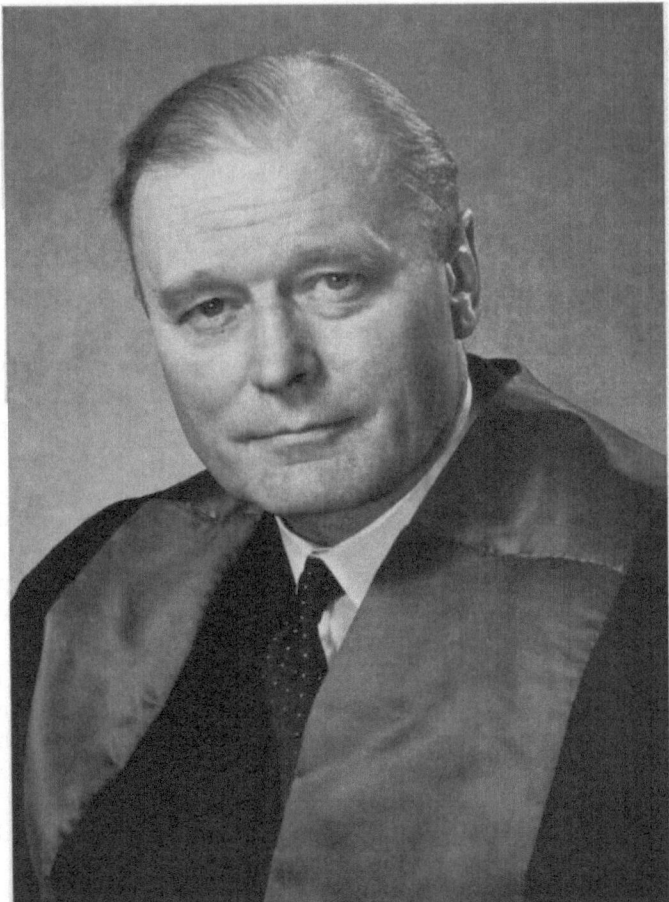

Plate 4. Prof. Sir HEDLEY ATKINS, K. B. E.

patients were premenopausal and had tumours which had taken many years to grow and become disseminated. In each case, he noted a response and the tumour deposits decreased in size or disappeared.

In 1895, when these operations were performed, the theory of the bacterial basis of disease was widely accepted. Cancer was thought to be due to so called "cancer bodies"—parasitic, intra-cellular organisms which were believed to cause the cellular activity and proliferation characteristic of malignant growth. BEATSON himself did not subscribe to this theory and preferred the unorthodox view that these intra-cellular bodies were simply products of cell breakdown and degeneration:

"I have felt for sometime, that the parasitic theory of cancer is an unsatisfactory one in many ways and that in directing all our energies to working it out we are losing time and searching for what will never be found, simply because it does not exist."

At this time, the function of the breast and particularly that of lactation was believed to be under nervous control. Earlier in his life, whilst working for his

M. D. Thesis, Beatson had studied lactation in the sheep and had formed the opinion that one organ might influence the secretion of another organ without direct nervous control. He described his idea in what must be one of the first direct references to the action of hormones:

"I am satisfied that in the ovary of the female and the testicle of the male, we have organs that send out influences more subtle and more mysterious that those emanating from the nervous system."

With remarkable foresight he went on to suggest that the ovaries might be the seat of the cause of carcinoma of the breast.

These were highly original and contentious thoughts and, although "ovariotomy" was frequently practised, its use under these circumstances seemed so outrageous that it led Beatson to anticipate criticism and even condemnation. He ended his paper by pleading that he had "been activated solely by the motives that guide all of us in the exercise of our profession; primarily, the interests of those who place themselves under our care and secondarily, the progress and advancement of the healing art."

There was no condemnation, nor even a word of comment. This singular description of how the growth of a malignant tumour could be influenced by treatment other than direct surgery was ignored. Beatson's paper was not accompanied by a leading article or annotation, nor was there any correspondence on the subject in ensuing copies of the Lancet.

And yet the point that oophorectomy could favourably affect the progress of advanced breast cancer had obviously been taken—probably because any therapy, however extraordinary, was worth trying for a condition that was otherwise untreatable. Within one year, further cases were being described to the East Anglian Branch of the British Medical Association and within two years, another report had appeared in the literature (Herman, 1898). By 1900, Stanley Boyd of the Charing Cross Hospital, was able to collect from various surgeons fifty-four cases of oophorectomy in advanced breast cancer. He reported that about one third responded (a figure that has not changed over the years) and stated that he was looking for methods to predict which patients would respond. We are still looking.

During the ensuing few years several further series appeared in the literature. The operation appears to have been confined to the treatment of advanced cases and its use as prophylaxis at mastectomy did not come until much later. Meanwhile, X-rays had been discovered and were developed, and it was not long before therapeutic doses of radiation were applied to the ovaries as a method of castration. By 1905, De Courmelles was irradiating the ovaries of patients with advanced breast cancer. In 1922, he described to the French Academie des Sciences, the advantages of a combined approach in the treatment of the locally advanced disease. He advised that both the tumour and the ovaries should be irradiated and mentioned two patients who had survived fifteen years following this treatment. In 1926, he reported that the response to ovarian irradiation was similar to that obtained by surgical ablation. The merits of the two methods of eliminating ovarian function are still being compared and debated.

In the early 1930's, natural and synthetic steroids became available and were investigated as treatment for the advanced disease. In 1939, Ulrich described two patients with breast cancer who had remissions following treatment with testosterone, and further reports on larger series were soon in the literature. There was no agreement on the value of androgens as therapy and indeed, one of the earliest reports might have persuaded surgeons not to pursue their use. FARROW and WOODARD (1942) described the changes in serum calcium levels than can follow the injection of testosterone propionate in patients with metastatic deposits in bones. They believed that the hormone stimulated the metastatic growth causing the ensuing hypercalc- aemia, and they suggested that this effect contra-indicated the use of androgens in treatment. Further studies did not endorse this suggestion, and androgens were soon accepted as treatment for the advanced disease.

In 1944, HADDOW and his colleagues, reported on a series of seventy three patients with primary cancers at many sites who had been treated with synthetic oestrogens. Triphenylchlorethylene, tryphenylmethylethylene and stilboestrol were used, and cancer of both the breast and prostate responded to the therapy. Stilb- oestrol proved to be the most active compound and was soon accepted as the drug of choice in the treatment of advanced breast cancer in post menopausal women.

In the mid 1940's it was believed that the benefit resulting from manipulation of the hormonal environment in patients with advanced breast cancer was largely due to the interruption of oestrogen synthesis. Certainly, removal of the ovaries had this effect. It was further possible that the failure of some patients to respond to this operation and the reason why a remission was inevitably followed by further cancerous growth might be due to the secretion of oestrogens by the adrenal glands. Cortisone was not available at this time and it was appreciated that to attempt to remove this further source of oestrogen by total adrenalectomy inevitably would be followed by death of the patient in Addisonian crisis. In 1947 and 1948 ATKINS tried to overcome this problem by removing all but a very small part of one adrenal. He performed the operation of sub-total adrenalectomy on six patients, removing one adrenal completely and three-quarters to seven-eighths of the other. (ATKINS, 1966). Two patients showed some measure of improvement, but he soon abandoned the operation, feeling that the margin of safety was too narrow and the degree of benefit too small.

When effective replacement therapy became available, CHARLES HUGGINS in Chicago became interested in the value of bilateral adrenalectomy in the manage- ment of prostatic cancer. Success in this field caused him to turn his attention to breast carcinoma, and 1952 HUGGINS and BERGENSTAL described the first successful total adrenalectomies in patients with the advanced disease. A year later, LUFT and OLIVECRONA (1953) described how a similar degree of remission could be obtained by removal of the pituitary gland. They carried out their hypophysectomies by a transfrontal approach and found this a safe and effective procedure with adequate cortisone cover. The operation had to be carried out by a neurosurgeon familiar with the technique and was beyond the scope of many units dealing with breast cancer. Other approaches to the pituitary fossa were explored and in 1955, FORREST and PEEBLES-BROWN described how the pituitary could be destroyed by the implantation of Radon seeds. This maneuvre could be performed by a general surgeon and re- sulted in very little upset to the patient. Unfortunately, Radon did not prove a satisfactory source of radiation. There was a high incidence of visual loss, third nerve paralysis and rhinorrhea and the degree of pituitary necrosis was variable. Further attempts at pituitary implantation were made using seeds of radioactive gold

(198 Au) but in therapeutic doses the gamma emission from this isotope also caused damage to structures around the pituitary gland. Eventually 90 Yttrium was found to be the most suitable source of radiation. 90 Yttrium is solely a beta emitter and has a short half life (2.4 days). Usually, two rods are placed in the gland using a canula introduced through the nose; providing the rods are accurately placed, there is little morbidity.

More recently hypophysectomy by the transphenoidal route (WESTOVER, RAND and GREENFIELD, 1960) has been advocated and may have advantages over both the other methods. The technique involves a dual approach to the gland through the nose and through an incision at the inner canthus of the eye. When the operation is performed by an Ear Nose and Throat surgeon, experienced in the technique, the whole gland can be removed in under one hour and with little upset to the patient.

In 1955, NISSEN-MEYER of Oslo suggested that oral cortisone therapy, combined with ovarian ablation, might effect a remission in some patients. He suggested that the treatment might accomplish a "medical adrenalectomy" and obviate the necessity for surgical removal of the adrenals and ovaries. Unfortunately this has not proved the case, although the treatment has found a place in the management of patients with the advanced disease who are unfit for adrenalectomy or hypophysectomy.

The ensuing chapters describe some of the research into hormones and human breast cancer that has been done in the past fifteen years — the period following this brief review. For convenience sake, history has been deemed to end and the present to begin in the early 1950s.

References

ATKINS, H. J. B.: Carcinoma of the breast. Ann. roy. Coll. Surg. Engl. **38**, 133 (1966).

BEATSON, G. W.: On the treatment of inoperable cases of carcinoma of the mamma: suggestions for a new method of treatment with illustrative cases. Lancet **1896 II**, 104, 162.

BOYD, S.: On oophorectomy in cancer of the breast. Brit. med. J. **1900 II**, 1161.

DE COURMELLES, F.: La radiothérapie combinée du sein et des ovaires contre les tumeurs du sein. C. R. Acad. Sci. (Paris) **174**, 503 (1922).

— Les rayons X et le radium en therapeutique gynecologique. Acta radiol. (Stockh.) **6**, 322 (1926).

FARROW, J. H., WOODARD, H. Q.: Influence of androgenic and oestrogenic substances on serum calcium in cases of skeletal metastases from breast cancer. J. Amer. med. Ass. **118**, 339 (1942).

FORREST, A. P. M., PEEBLES BROWN, D. A.: Pituitary-radon implant for breast cancer. Lancet **1955 I**, 1054.

FOULDS, L.: Mammary tumours in hybrid mice: growth and progressive of spontaneous tumours. Brit. J. Cancer **3**, 345 (1949).

HADDOW, A. L.: Nature (Lond.) **136**, 868 (1935).

— WATKINSON, J. M., PATERSON, E., KOLLER, P. C.: Influence of synthetic oestrogens upon advanced malignant disease. Brit. med. J. **1944 II**, 393.

HERMAN, G. E.: Lancet **1898 I**, 1612.

HUGGINS, C.: Experimental mammary cancer; induction and extinction. Symposium on the prognosis of malignant tumours of the breast. Basel-New York: S. Karger 1963.

— BERGENSTAL, D. M.: Inhibition of human mammary and prostatic cancers by adrenalectomy. Cancer Res. **12**, 134 (1952).

KORTEWEG, R., THOMAS, F.: Tumor induction and tumor growth in hypophysectomised mice. Amer. J. Cancer **37**, 36 (1939).

LACCASAGNE, A.: Apparition de Cancer de la Mamelle chez la Souris mâle, Soumis à des Injections de Folliculine. C. R. Acad. Sci. (Paris) 195, 630 (1932).

LOEB, L.: Further investigations on the origin of tumors in mice. VI. Internal secretions as a factor in the origin of tumors. J. med. Res. XL, 477 (1919—1920).

LUFT, R., OLIVECRONA, H.: Experiences with hypophysectomy in man. J. Neurosurg. 10, 301 (1953).

MURRAY, W. S.: Ovarian secretion and tumour incidence. J. Cancer Res. 12, 18 (1928).

NISSEN-MEYER, R.: Cancer Mammae: Forsok med en ny endokrinologisk behandlings-kombinasjon. Nord. Med. 53, 186 (1955).

SCHINZINGER, A.: Über carcinoma mammae. Zentr.-Org. ges. Chir. 29, 55 (1899).

SHIMKIN, M. B., WYMAN, R. S.: Effect of adrenalectomy and ovariectomy on mammary carcinogenesis in Strain C_3H mice. J. nat. Cancer Inst. 6, 187 (1945).

ULRICH, P.: Testosterone (hormone male) et son role possible dans la traitement de certain cancers du sein. Acta Un. int. Cancer 4, 377 (1939).

WESTOVER, J. L., RAND, R. W., GREENFIELD, M. A.: Yttrium-90 transnasal hypophysectomy: technic and dosimetry. Radiology 74, 86 (1960).

Chapter 2

The Ovaries

Castration is the oldest endocrine treatment for breast cancer. Many well documented accounts of its use are now in the literature (see for instance, ADAIR et al., 1945; DOUGLAS, 1952; TREVES and FINKBEINER, 1958; TAYLOR, 1962) and there are also several extensive reviews. LEWISON (1962) has contributed a detailed and thoughtful account of the comparative merits of prophylactic and therapeutic castration in which much of the available world literature is reviewed. Other valuable reviews have come from LEWISON (1965) and NISSEN-MEYER (1965).

Two workers have been responsible for almost all the prospective clinical investigations. MARY COLE (1964, 1968), originally working with PATERSON and RUSSELL at the Christie Hospital in Manchester, has carried out the only large randomised trial on the value of prophylactic castration. And ROAR NISSEN-MEYER (1965, 1967), of the Norwegian Radium Hospital in Oslo, has undertaken trials to assess the value of castration in pre- and post-menopausal women, and to compare the merits of ovarian irradiation and oophorectomy.

The emphasis throughout has been on five questions:
1. What part does castration play in the treatment of the advanced disease?
2. What part does castration play as a prophylactic measure after mastectomy?
3. Is castration better carried out prophylactically or therapeutically?
4. Is surgical castration preferable to ovarian irradiation?
5. What are the physiological results of castration?

None of these questions has been satisfactorily answered, but the evidence so far has enabled some conclusions to be drawn, even though absolute proof of these conclusions has not yet been obtained.

1. Castration in the Advanced Disease

a) Response

No endocrine treatment, either by hormone administration or by ablation, has ever been known to cure a patient with breast cancer. This is irrespective of whether the cancer has spread locally or distantly. Where treatment by conventional surgical methods is not possible, the principal aim of endocrine therapy in the advanced disease must be to palliate. In this context, palliation means not only the alleviation of distressing symptoms but also the reduction in size or the disappearance of active lesions. The resulting benefit can be so pronounced that the patient is restored to normal health for several years.

Castration need not be artificially induced to do this. The occurrence of the natural menopause in a patient who has carcinoma of the breast can cause the tumour to regress. SMITHERS (1952, 1953), reported three patients who had marked regression of the primary tumour following the natural menopause. But the menopause seldom occurs at the moment when it would be most helpful to a patient with breast cancer and so has to be induced artificially, either by surgical removal of the ovaries or by ovarian irradiation.

There are many conflicting reports of the remission rate that can be expected following castration. Principally this is because there has been no measure of agreement between various workers and centres on the criteria of a successful response. Indeed, in some reports, the criteria of response have not even been mentioned. NISSEN-MEYER (1965), in his monograph on castration in female breast cancer, listed fifteen series, including a total of 2,221 patients, in which the remission rate varied between 15.2 per cent and 50 per cent. Such a variation could not be the result of different techniques of castration, nor of differences in the patient material available to each investigator. More likely, it is because each assessment was related to different criteria of success. Some physicians were satisfied that a response had occurred when the growth of a few lesions was retarded and there was relief from pain. Others required evidence that all lesions had diminished in size and that no new lesions had occurred — albeit for a very short time. Still others imposed a time limit on success and refused to accept a period of remission of less than six months.

Under these circumstances, it is impossible to say what is correct and what is incorrect. There is no right or wrong when a whole range of equally valid possibilities and variables is considered. Each worker has to choose his own criteria and be able to defend his choice.

There are two rules which most workers have adhered to in these investigations and about which there can be little controversy. Firstly, only objective evidence of remission should be accepted. This is not to infer that subjective remission, such as the relief of pain, is not important — particularly to the patient — but subjective remission can be so greatly affected by factors other than the treatment under test that its use as a measurement of response is quite unreliable. For example, relief from pain can be the result of enforced bed rest; apparent improvement in the patient's appearance and well-being can be due to hospitalisation and good nursing; even the enthusiastic application of a new treatment can cause the patient to say she feels better. The decision that a remission has occurred must depend solely on the measureable improvement of lesions which can be either seen, palpated or demonstrated radiologically. These measurements should have been carried out at regular intervals and, on each occasion, compared both with the measurements taken at the previous examination and with the condition of the patient before treatment was applied.

Secondly, the criteria of response, which an observer accepts as proof of remission, must be declared with his results. These criteria should not be ambiguous, should be applicable to every case, and no exception should be made unless the reason is clearly stated.

It would be preferable to have an agreed set of rules for the assessment of palliative treatments for patients with advanced breast cancer. In 1965, an International

Symposium was held to try to formulate such a set of rules. This did not prove possible at the time, but the Symposium at least made workers from many centres state exactly how they assessed the response of their patients. The report of the Symposium (HAYWARD and BULBROOK, 1966) described a few well-defined protocols.

An overall remission rate for ovarian ablation cannot be agreed without an accepted definition of remission, nor can a comparison between the results of two centres be accepted unless their protocols are identical (it is doubtful even then if such an exercise is worthwhile, considering the major differences that can occur in patient material). Therefore, after consideration of the world literature, the presumption of an overall percentage remission following castration can have only a restricted meaning. NISSEN-MEYER (1965) in analysing a collected series of 2,221 patients, stated that 29.29 per cent experienced a remission. LEWISON (1962) concluded his review on prophylactic and therapeutic castration by stating ... "A review of the clinical results of therapeutic castration in pre-menopausal women with advanced breast cancer, indicates that oophorectomy is an effective palliative procedure in about 25 per cent of the patients."

The surgeon, who wishes to know his patient's chances of success, can accept these figures, but must understand the limits of the evidence on which they are based. Much of this difficulty could be avoided if there was an accepted international protocol for the assessment of response to the palliative treatment of advanced breast cancer — and there is a great need for this.

Table 1 shows details of 1,259 patients included in five reports of therapeutic castration. The remission rates vary from 15.2 per cent to 47.5 per cent—a three-fold difference. The reason for this difference can easily be seen: firstly, the material differs—for instance the proportions of pre- and post-menopausal women vary from series to series; secondly, the criteria of assessment are never the same—some observers insist that all lesions regress, some that only the dominant lesions should regress, some do not specify; thirdly, the time that this regression lasts before the treatment is considered successful is often not given; fourthly, some include subjective remission in their assessment, some exclude it.

Surely there could be some measure of agreement on this, if only for the purpose of reporting. The protocol of the Co-operative Breast Cancer Group (1966) probably has most to offer and, with a few modifications, stands the best chance of general acceptance. A just criticism is that it does not specify a lower time limit during which a patient has to be in remission before a treatment is considered successful. This allows too much latitude in its use, but the protocol was designed specifically to evaluate the response rate of patients given experimental synthetic steroids, and few amendments would be necessary to widen its application. At least it does state unequivocally what is or is not acceptable. Using an embryo form of this protocol, GORDON and SEGALOFF (1958) described their experience with surgical and x-ray castration and reported a 32.7 per cent remission rate. They studied only forty nine patients, and there must be some doubt whether this remission rate represents that which might be found in a larger series, but it would be encouraging to hear of other series analysed in a similar way—perhaps using the Breast Cancer Group's present protocol.

In a nicely analysed study of 354 regularly menstruating patients, FRACCHIA et al. (1969) found that 34.5 per cent had an objective remission; in those patients who

Table 1. *Details of five published reports on therapeutic castration*

Author	Patient material	No. of patients	Criteria of assessment	Time limit of response	Type of response	Per cent remission
ADAIR et al., 1945	Mixed therapeutic and prophylactic. Pre- and postmenopausal	335 (248 advanced)	Response assessed on survival time only. Clinical benefit mentioned when known	Survival must be more than 2 years	Subjective and objective	15.2
DOUGLAS, 1952	Pre- and postmenopausal	175	Regression or disappearance of all soft tissue lesions. Calcification at bone deposits or relief of bone pain	None	Subjective and objective	20.6
KENNEDY and FORTUNY, 1964	170 patients premenopausal + 7 patients within 5 years postmenopausal with positive smears	177	Calcification of bone metastases, or tumour masses decreased in size by 25% or more — unknown whether all lesions have to respond	None	Objective only	47.5
TAYLOR, 1962	Premenopausal or within 1 year postmenopausal. Analysis only of those who survived oophorectomy by 1 month	381	Measurable decrease in size of one or more foci (clinical or radiological) without new lesions occurring or progression of existing lesions	6 months sustained remission	Objective only	29.7
TREVES and FINKBEINER, 1958	Pre- and postmenopausal. Also post-ovarian irradiation (14 cases)	191	Measurable evidence of remission of major lesions (not stated whether all have to improve) in bone or soft tissues	None (although duration of remission stated for each case)	Objective only	37.0

were irregularly menstruating, only 27.3 per cent responded. FRACCHIA and his colleagues employed very strict criteria of response and included only those patients in whom all lesions had improved for at least 6 months. Their response rate would be accepted by most workers in this field.

At the present, castration is considered the first choice of treatment for premenopausal patients with advanced breast cancer who are unsuitable for local radiotherapy of surgery.

b) Prediction

Whatever may be the merits of castration as a palliative measure in advanced breast cancer, there are many who feel that it is worthwhile, if only for it's reputed value in predicting a patient's subsequent response to adrenalectomy or hypophysectomy. If a good response is obtained from castration, there may be a favourable response to major ablation. Conversely, if no benefit is derived from castration, some workers consider hypophysectomy or adrenalectomy is not worth doing. Undoubtedly, this again begs the question of what exactly is meant by a good response to castration; but nevertheless there have been many reports of a positive correlation between the results of castration and the results of subsequent endocrine therapy, and presumably most observers at least judge the remissions of their own patients in a standard way, even if they cannot compare their results with those of others. HALL et al. (1963) described sixty nine patients who had a favourable response to surgical castration. 23 per cent of these subsequently responded to hormone therapy. Of their 213 patients who failed to respond to castration, only 7 per cent benefited from hormone therapy. MACDONALD (1957) found that 44.7 per cent of forty eight patients who had had an objective remission following castration, subsequently had a successful response to adrenalectomy or hypophysectomy. Out of 71 patients who failed to respond to castration, 11.3 had a subsequent remission from adrenalectomy or hypophysectomy.

Other workers have not found the results of castration so useful. DAO and NEMOTO (1965) reported that the response to surgical castration showed some correlation with the subsequent response to adrenalectomy, but later (DAO, NEMOTO and BROSS, 1968) concluded that castration failure did not necessarily infer that adrenalectomy would also fail. Similarly, MOORE et al. (1968) found the response to oophorectomy unreliable as a method of predicting the response to subsequent major ablative procedures. Both MOORE et al. (1968) and FAIRGRIEVE (1965) have commented that, in practice, castration response is rarely available as a criterion (see page 54).

Nevertheless, although the prediction of response to hormone therapy, as described by HALL et al. (1963), has little clinical application (it is just as simple in practice to try drugs), any treatment which gives some forecast of the subsequent response to adrenalectomy or hypophysectomy, is almost worthwhile considering on that merit alone. What may prove interesting is whether assays of endocrine function (see pages 57—66) and the response to castration give similar information in predicting the response to adrenalectomy or hypophysectomy. From the use of hormone assays, patients can be selected who will stand up to a 40 per cent chance of responding to subsequent major ablation. The question remains whether this method of prediction selects the same patients as castration or whether the two methods are complementary to one another and, if applied together, would enable a much more accurate forecast to be made than is obtained from either alone.

HAYWARD and BULBROOK (1968) have described a study in which this problem is under investigation. All premenopausal patients with advanced breast cancer have hormone assays carried out on a 24-hour urine specimen; an oophorectomy is then performed. If, after at least six weeks, no response is noted to the oophorectomy, a further 24-hour urine specimen is collected and the assays repeated. Providing the patient is still fit, a hypophysectomy is then performed, either by the transphenoidal or by the transfrontal route. Should the oophorectomy result in a remission, then no further treatment is undertaken whilst that remission lasts. Eventually, when the disease again progresses, the hormone excretion is measured once more and a hypophysectomy performed. From this investigation, data should be available on the relationship between the response to oophorectomy and the measure of endocrine function on the one hand, and the subsequent response to hypophysectomy on the other.

c) Adjunctive Therapy

Little progress has been made in evaluating supplementary agents which could enhance the effect of castration in the treatment of the advanced disease. It may be remembered that BEATSON's (1896) original patients were both prescribed thyroid in addition to having their ovaries removed. HERMAN (1900) emphasised the value of thyroid as supplementary therapy to oophorectomy and re-analysed BOYD's (1900) data to show that there was a higher incidence of remission in those patients who had received thyroid in addition to having their ovaries removed, compared with those who had had only an oophorectomy. More recently, LOESER (1954) spent much of his life, championing the cause of thyroid treatment for breast cancer, but found little support. On two occasions, LEMON (1957, 1959) has described patients previously castrated who in addition have been given either dessicated thyroid or triiodothyronine. His cases were treated principally with cortisone or prednisone and the thyroid was used to prevent myxoedema and to produce further inhibition of the pituitary. But Lemon suggests that thyroid therapy may produce prolonged remissions by minimising the side effects of cortisone treatment and reinforcing the tumour suppressive action of cortisone. LEWISON (1962) described a trial by the Cooperative Breast Group of the Cancer Chemotherapy National Service Centre where two groups of castrated patients are compared. One group is receiving thyroid as adjunctive therapy, and the other is receiving a placebo; the choice is made by random sample. No results of this trial are yet available. Until there is further evidence of the effect of thyroid treatment there seems little justification in it's routine administration to patients who have been castrated.

The use of corticosteroids with castration, in the treatment of the advanced disease, has a marked therapeutic effect and this will be dealt with in Chapter 6.

Little work has been done on the combined effect of castration and androgen administration. Both of these measures act principally on premenopausal patients, both have approximately the same effect, and yet they probably act in different ways. If used together they might well give a better response than either used separately.

Castration as a Prophylactic Measure

Although the word "prophylactic" is used to describe the place of castration in the treatment of early breast cancer, it is a misnomer. Castration is used in the hope that the patient's prognosis can be improved. In effect, the best that can be achieved is that, if the carcinoma had already spread beyond the bounds of the primary operation, the appearance of metastatic deposits can be delayed. This delay means that the period free from overt disease may be increased, and possibly—but not necessarily—there will be a similar improvement in survival. The metastatic deposits will always appear eventually and there is no question of permanent destruction of the remaining cancer cells. If the primary operation has been incomplete, castration can never do more than postpone the inevitable recurrence of the cancer.

The principal question to be answered is how efficient is castration in accomplishing this postponement. Is its efficiency so great and the degree or benefit obtained so worthwhile that it should be performed on all patients, or is the number of patients in whom the course of the disease is effectively altered only a small proportion of the whole; so small in fact, that the castration of the many cannot be justified for so little a return?

There can be little doubt that the cessation of rhythmical ovarian function can delay the appearance of metastatic carcinoma in those patients whose disease recurs after mastectomy. The natural menopause can probably accomplish this if it occurs at the right time. WAGONER et al. (1967) investigated the mortality from breast cancer among teachers and administrative staffs of Roman Catholic Sisterhoods in the United States. They noted a break in the mortality curve at the time of the menopause. Also, LEWISON (1962) describes a discussion published in the supplement of a report of the Committee on Research by the American Medical Association, where it was noted that when the natural menopause occurred prior to the onset of secondaries, the free interval (described in this context as the time from primary treatment to the start of palliative hormone therapy) was markedly increased. This was a retrospective study and there may have been other variables involved, but nevertheless, it does seem that the natural menopause, if it occurs after the mastectomy and before the appearance of secondaries, has a suppressing effect on the growth of cancer tissue.

An artificial menopause, induced either by surgical castration or by destroying ovarian function with X-irradiation, probably has the same effect as the natural menopause. A few patients will have recurrence of their carcinoma delayed but it is not known exactly how many will benefit.

COLE (1964, 1968) has undertaken a clinical trial on the value of an x-ray induced menopause in the management of early breast cancer. From 1948 to 1955 all patients (premenopausal or within two years of the menopause), other than those whose disease was so advanced that hormone therapy was the only rational treatment, were randomly divided into two groups. The patients in one group had an artificial menopause by the administration of 450 r to the mid pelvis, using 250 KV x-rays. The patients in the second group did not receive ovarian irradiation—otherwise the treatment of the two groups was the same. These groups were not comprised solely of patients who were immediately post-mastectomy. Some had had their mastectomy some time previously and the disease had already recurred, whilst others were presenting for the first time with an inoperable breast carcinoma. Nevertheless, these patients represented a small fraction of the total and COLE was able to report on 596 patients (293 irradiated and 303 controls) who were post mastectomy and in whom the disease had not recurred at the time of randomisation.

Table 2 shows the survival of these patients ten years after operation; although there was a higher proportion surviving in the treatment group than in the control group, the difference was not statistically significant. The greatest improvement in

Table 2. *Comparison of survival in treatment and control groups 10 years after prophylactic castration* (COLE, 1968)

Number of cases		Crude survival %		P
Irradiated	Control	Irradiated	Control	
293	303	54.9	47.5	0.07

Table 3. *Comparison of survival in treatment and control groups 10 years after prophylactic castration related to axillary node involvement.* (COLE, 1968)

	Number of cases		Crude survival %		P
	Irradiated	Control	Irradiated	Control	
Axillary nodes not involved	90	103	80.0	68.0	0.06
Axillary nodes involved	203	200	43.8	37.0	0.16

Table 4. *Comparison of incidence of recurrence in treatment and control groups 10 years after prophylactic castration* (COLE, 1968)

	Number of cases		Incidence %		P
	Irradiated	Control	Irradiated	Control	
Recurrence breast area (including axillary and supraclavicular nodes)	293	303	23.2	29.7	0.07
Distant metastases	—	—	46.1	54.5	0.04

survival occurred in those patients whose axillary nodes were not involved at mastectomy (Table 3). When the incidence of distant metastases was compared, a difference was shown between the treated and control groups which achieved formal statistical significance (Table 4).

The trial has already been widely quoted and to many it has seemed surprising and disappointing that the benefit achieved by castration at mastectomy proved so slight. Although nearly 300 castrated patients were followed for ten years, the improvement in survival and in the incidence of distant metastases was marginal. But COLE's results may not be truly representative of the benefit that can be achieved. Castration was effected by radiotherapy, and the dosage employed was only 450 r. This dose of radiation may not be sufficient to obtain complete cessation of ovarian function, especially in young people. Indeed, 33 per cent of COLE's patients aged under 40 had a return of menstrual bleeding after treatment. Nowadays, a higher dose of radiation would be used (about 2,000 rads).

ROAR NISSEN-MEYER (1965, 1967) has also undertaken randomised controlled clinical trials to test the value of primary ovarian ablation. To understand his results, it is important to appreciate the principles he followed before he included a patient in his trials. These principles were complicated, and he ended up with rather special groups of patients on which he made his comparison. It is worth studying his protocol in some detail.

Premenopausal patients were entered into the trial only if he considered their prognosis was good. If the patient had a bad prognosis, he felt he could not justify her being randomised between the treatment and control groups. All patients in this category (i. e. premenopausal and with a poor risk) were not included in the trial and were electively castrated.

It is not quite clear what were his exact criteria for judging the prognosis of his patients after mastectomy, although tumour size, grade, and axillary node involvement were certainly taken into account. Because of this selection, only 161 premenopausal patients—those he considered had a good prognosis—were available for analysis.

All postmenopausal patients were entered into the trial. When the study was started, he did not expect castration would benefit postmenopausal patients and therefore did not feel bound to recommend the treatment if the prognosis seemed poor. In effect, a considerable difference was noted between the results in the treated and control groups in his postmenopausal women, and this part of the trial was stopped when 175 patients had been included. Because there was no selection on the grounds of prognosis, his trial on postmenopausal women included many patients with more advanced disease and more malignant tumours than his trial on premenopausal women. After randomisation, the patients in his treatment groups either had an oophorectomy or had their ovaries irradiated. The patients in his control groups had their ovaries left intact.

Table 5. *Proportions surviving and free from disease 5 years after prophylactic castration.* (NISSEN-MEYER, 1965)

	Treated	Control
Crude survival at 5 years (%)	78.3	67.3
Free from disease at 5 years (%)	72.4	59.0

His results were analysed differently to COLE's (1968) but, nevertheless, there were points of similarity. In his premenopausal patients, there was no statistical difference in the crude survival rate between treated patients and controls—in fact, more patients died in the treatment group (although this was largely accounted for by deaths from other causes). However, the cumulative rates free from disease favoured the treatment group, although it was felt that the observation time was too short for a valid conclusion to be made.

The comparison between the treatment and control groups in his postmenopausal patients is shown in Table 5. The maximum differences between the groups, both in the numbers free from disease and in the crude survival rate, occurred during the

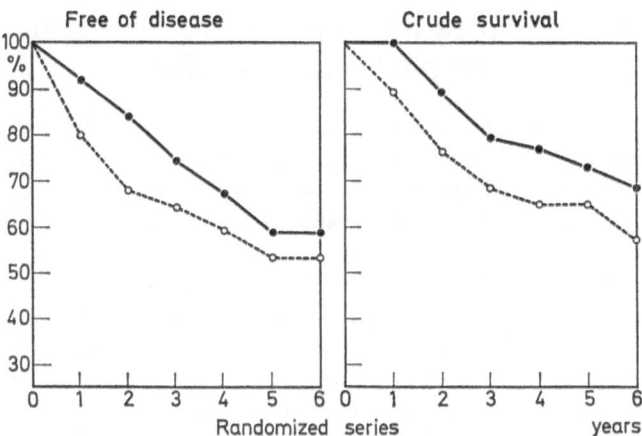

Fig. 1. Recurrence and survival experience in treated postmenopausal women and in controls (NISSEN-MEYER, 1965; reproduced with permission). ●————● With primary castration (88 cases); o– – –o Without primary castration (86 cases)

first two years after treatment (Fig. 1) and this difference was statistically significant. NISSEN-MEYER summarised his conclusions as follows:

... "The favourable effect of postoperative ovarian irradiation on both recurrence-free period and survival was established with a high degree of certainty in postmenopausal patients... In the Norwegian Radium Hospital, we now give primary ovarian irradiation to postmenopausal patients up to the age of seventy years."

These results are difficult to interpret. Firstly, the comparison of the treated and control groups in premenopausal patients, whom most physicians believe benefit from ovarian ablation after mastectomy, gave inconclusive results—probably because of the high degree of patient selection. Secondly, the trial on postmenopausal patients, whom few consider likely to benefit from ovarian irradiation, showed a considerable and significant advantage to those treated—at least during the first few years.

This finding has not yet been confirmed. Indeed, FRACCHIA et al. (1969) showed that only 3.5 per cent of 85 postmenopausal women with the advanced disease who were therapeutically castrated had an objective remission — and all of these were within one year of the menopause.

It is not possible to make a direct comparison between NISSEN-MEYER's and COLE's results. Not only is the presentation of the results different, but also the composition of the two series and the methods of ovarian ablation are dissimilar. Many of NISSEN-MEYER's patients had an oophorectomy performed, and those that were castrated by irradiation received a higher dose of x-rays than the patients in COLE's series (it was estimated that NISSEN-MEYER's patients received 1,000 r to each ovary).

Nevertheless, it can be concluded from both COLE's and NISSEN-MEYER's series that ovarian ablation, performed immediately after mastectomy, can effect some benefit to the patient, in terms of both survival and period free from recurrence.

The Comparative Values of Therapeutic and Prophylactic Castration

At least one attempt has been made to compare directly the results of prophylactic castration with the results of therapeutic castration. KENNEDY, MIELKE and FORTUNY (1964) compared 108 patients, undergoing prophylactic castration, with 105 patients undergoing therapeutic castration. The two series of patients were homogeneous in respect to age, stage and castration technique. They concluded that the time interval between initial tumour therapy and recurrence was longer in the prophylactic group (38.2 months compared with 24.6 months), but the interval from recurrence to death was longer in the therapeutic group (13.7 months to 23.4 months). When the two periods were considered together, the mean interval from initial tumour therapy to death was similar in the two groups.

KENNEDY and his colleagues' two groups were not randomised and, in spite of the matching, were not strictly comparable. For instance, they could make no allowance for the fact that the patients in the therapeutic castration group must have had slowly growing tumours for castration to be possible. In a significant proportion of patients, the cancer recurs and progresses so quickly that elective treatment cannot be carried out. These patients would not be included in the therapeutic group but would have been included in the prophylactic group where castration was performed before the disease recurred.

Elsewhere, KENNEDY (1964) summarised his findings by stating . . . "It is strongly concluded that late therapeutic castration is the preferable procedure in employing the technique of castration."

In reality, the choice between prophylactic and therapeutic castration has not been settled. LEWISON (1962) in his general review of the merits of the two procedures, could only conclude that the matter would not be resolved until a controlled clinical experiment had been undertaken in which the method of castration was determined by random sample. Since this was written, the results of COLE's (1964, 1968) and NISSEN-MEYER's (1965, 1967) trials have been reported, but the subject is still debated and there is still controversy.

In practice, there are three possible ways of using castration:

(i) All patients can be castrated after mastectomy in the knowledge that a few will have a longer period free from recurrence and possibly a longer survival.

(ii) Castration can be carried out only on those patients whose disease has recurred, in the hope that some of them will have a reasonable remission from their symptoms and that this remission may continue for some years; but knowing that this recurrence might have been manifest later had a prophylactic castration been performed.

(iii) An attempt may be made to select patients for either treatment.

Medical opinion is divided almost equally on (i) and (ii). Numerous articles have reviewed the problem and, on the basis of personal experience or collected cases, the authors have opted either in favour of prophylactic castration (SMITH and SMITH, 1953; ALRICH, LIDDLE and MORTON, 1957; TREVES, 1957; ROSENBERG and UHLMANN, 1959; RENNAES, 1960) or against it (TAYLOR, 1939; ADAIR et al., 1945; HUCK, 1952; McWHIRTER, 1956).

Option (iii) raises the question of whether it is possible to be selective at the present. Can patients be identified on whom prophylactic castration should be carried out, and others who should not be treated at mastectomy but only if the disease recurs? The ideal circumstances can easily be defined. Therapeutic castration should be performed only on those patients whose tumour has recurred and will be responsive—a situation which is partly identifiable. Prophylactic castration should be performed only on those patients whose tumour *will* recur and be responsive—at the present there is no precise way of detecting these patients.

In practice, the choice between treatments can be influenced by many factors, and the emphasis which is placed on each factor may vary in different clinic and from patient to patient.

The available evidence which may affect a decision can be summarised as follows:

a) For Prophylactic Castration

α) Prophylactic Castration Probably Gives a Small Improvement in Survival. Nissen-Meyer (1965, 1967) concluded that primary ovarian irradiation, in post-menopausal women up to the age of seventy years, had a favourable effect on survival. He also concluded that there was a trend in favour of primary ovarian in premenopausal women. Cole (1964, 1968) (in what was really a comparative trial between prophylactic and therapeutic castration as most of her control group were given a therapeutic castration if they recurred) concluded that a primary irradiation menopause increased the survival rate in operable breast cancer patients.

Similar conclusions have been reached in reviews of uncontrolled series. Smith and Smith (1953), Alrich et al. (1957), Treves (1957) and Rosenberg and Uhlmann (1959) all found that prophylactic castration increased survival. The overall improvement in the 5 year survival rate is probably about 5 per cent (Cole, 1964).

β) Prophylactic Castration Postpones the Onset of Recurrence. Cole (1968) showed that, compared with controls, appreciably less of her treated patients had distant metastases ten years after mastectomy. There was a similar but less marked effect on local recurrence.

Nissen-Meyer (1967) also noticed an increase in the period free from recurrence. The difference between his treated and control groups was most marked in post-menopausal patients with Stage 2 growths. Here, a significantly higher number of castrated patients were free from disease 1 and 2 years after mastectomy.

Kennedy et al. (1964) also inferred that the period from mastectomy to recurrence was nearly 14 months longer in castrated patients.

γ) Patients can be Selected for Prophylactic Mastectomy by the Spread or the Degree of Malignancy of their Tumour. For instance, only patients with high grade, high stage tumours may be treated. Moore et al. (1968) describe how they only treat patients with a medial lump or with a high chance of recurrence because of involved axillary lymph nodes.

δ) The Patients on whom Prophylactic Castration has no Effect, Obscure the Results in the Few that are Helped. The small overall increase in recurrence-free period and survival must be the result of considerable improvement experienced by the few whom the treatment affected favourably.

Nissen-Meyer (1967) has estimated the number of extra years free from disease enjoyed by patients not cured by mastectomy who receive prophylactic irradiation.

For his recurrence cases he has shown that the average time free from symptoms is prolonged by about 2 years in premenopausal women and 1—2 years in post-menopausal women.

ε) *Prophylactic Castration Prevents any Future Pregnancy*. Pregnancy is believed to be dangerous to women who have had a mastectomy for breast cancer—at least, if it occurs within a few years of the operation. Pregnancy can make no difference to a patient's cure but, when viable cancer tissue remains, it may accelerate the development of metastases. If castration is carried out, pregnancy would not be possible. On the other hand there are those who believe that pregnancy is beneficial after mastectomy. VERA PETERS (1968) has reported a series in which she compared the survival of mastectomy patients, who had subsequently become pregnant, with the survival of matched controls. She showed that the pregnant patients fared better than the controls and she now recommends pregnancy to her patients almost as a therapeutic measure.

b) For Therapeutic Castration

α) *Therapeutic Castration is Probably the most Effective Endocrine Treatment for Premenopausal Women with Recurrent Breast Cancer*. Approximately 25 per cent of them will obtain a worthwhile remission which may last several years. If a prophylactic castration had been performed this treatment would not be available.

β) *Patients Having a Therapeutic Castration may Survive Longer after Recurrence*. KENNEDY et al. (1964) estimated that the time from recurrence to death was 10 months longer in patients having a therapeutic castration than in those who had a prophylactic castration. On the other hand, NISSEN-MEYER (1967) concluded that the interval between recurrence and death was about the same.

γ) *Patients Castrated Therapeutically are those with Recurrent Disease and therefore known to be in need of Treatment*. With prophylactic therapy, many women will be needlessly castrated as their tumours have been completely extirpated at the primary operation and will not recur. It is difficult to know how many there are of these. The manifestations of recurrence of breast cancer are so protean that it is virtually impossible ever to be certain that a patient has been cured. In COLE's (1968) control group of 303 patients, 54.5 per cent had distant recurrence ten years after the primary operation (see Table 4). Possibly 60 per cent of patients treated for primary breast cancer eventually have a recurrence. Of these, about a quarter will have responsive tumours. This means that only 15 per cent of patients given a prophylactic castration will benefit and 85 per cent will be treated unnecessarily.

δ) *There is Some Evidence that the Introduction of Modern Endocrine Therapy has Negated the Value of Prophylactic Castration*. COLE (1964) has shown that the survival experience of her control group has improved in recent years. She presumes this is due to the recent introduction and use of hormone administration and ovarian ablation as treatment for the advanced case. Fig. 2 shows a comparison of her castrated and control groups for the periods 1948—1952 and 1953—1955. No apparent difference is seen in the mortality rate for the castrated groups in both periods but the mortality rate for the control group of 1953—1955 is less than that for 1948—1952. Table 6 shows that the percentage of patients in the control group treated by hormone administration or ablative procedures is almost double in the 1953—1955 period.

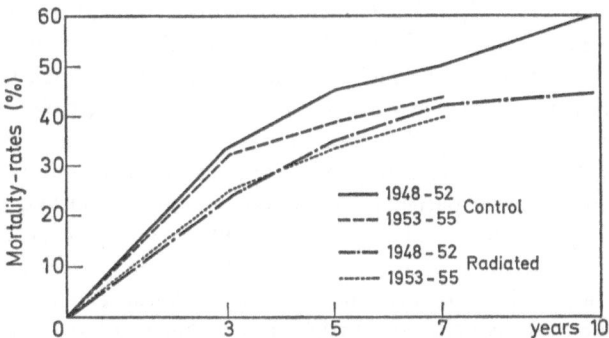

Fig. 2. Comparison of irradiation and control groups for periods 1948—1952 and 1953 to 1955 (COLE, 1964, reproduced with permission). ———— Control 1948—1952 (145 cases); — — — control 1953—1955 (160 cases); — — · — radiated 1948—1952 (144 cases); - - - - radiated 1953—1955 (149 cases)

Table 6. *Percentage of patients treated with hormonal procedures in 1948—1952 and 1953—1955.* (COLE, 1964)

	Number of cases		Percentage treated by hormonal procedures	
	Radiated	Control	Radiated	Control
1948—1952	144	145	14.6	15.2
1953—1955	147	155	19.8	31.8

ε) *The Result of Therapeutic Castration may Help in Predicting the Subsequent Response of a Patient to Adrenalectomy or Hypophysectomy.* On the other hand, NISSEN-MEYER (1965) points out that this is no reason for carrying out therapeutic as opposed to prophylactic castration because not all physicians use adrenalectomy or hypophysectomy in their management of the advanced disease. Also the response to therapeutic castration is not a very reliable guide to the response of subsequent ablation, and can be used in very few cases. MOORE et al. (1968) found that in only 9 per cent of all their patients, treated for secondary disease, was prior oophorectomy available as a criterion.

ζ) *Castration can Cause Malignant Deposits to Grow Faster* (WILSON et al., 1958). Occasional exacerbation of the cancer almost certainly follows both prophylactic and therapeutic castration but would be a particularly unfortunate consequence of the former procedure. Similar effects have been noted following androgen therapy (MYERS et al., 1956), oestrogen therapy (EMERSON and JESSIMAN, 1956) and adrenalectomy (WILSON et al., 1958). At present, no prediction can be made of which patients will be made worse, and this development is a serious hazard of all forms of endocrine therapy.

η) *Early Castration may Increase the Likelihood of a Woman Developing Ischaemic Heart Disease.* OLIVER and BOYD (1959) showed that the incidence of ischaemic heart disease was increased in women, aged 35 or under, who had had a bilateral oophorectomy. SZNAJDERMAN and OLIVER (1963) described similar findings in women who had had a premature spontaneous menopause. They also reported that, in postmenopausal women, serum lipid levels increased with the length of time which had elapsed since the menopause. However, NOVAK and WILLIAMS (1960) were unable to demonstrate a difference in the incidence of arteriosclerosis when they compared the findings at autopsy in castrated women and non-castrated controls.

In practice, a rational choice between the two treatments can seldom be made. Essentially, the only way to get a maximum response from prophylactic castration is to treat all premenopausal patients and—if NISSEN-MEYER's (1965, 1967) findings be confirmed—all postmenopausal patients as well. Some surgeons temporise and use prophylactic castration only in patients who have a high chance of recurrence. Many are unwilling even to do this. They regard the reward, in terms of improved recurrence and survival, as being too little for the number of patients who will be treated unnecessarily.

Castration will be an accepted therapy in the early disease only when those patients who will respond can be identified with certainty at mastectomy. Possibly, measurements of endocrine status will provide this information. Hormone assays have been shown to correlate with response to adrenalectomy and hypophysectomy (see pp. 57—66) and might also be used in predicting the results of castration.

A trial to investigate the relationship between endocrine function and the response to prophylactic castration has recently been reported by MEAKIN and his colleagues (1968) from the Princess Margaret Hospital in Toronto and the Imperial Cancer Research Fund in England.

One purpose of this trial is to repeat and amplify on the investigations made by COLE and NISSEN-MEYER. This will be done firstly by testing the value of an irradiation menopause using a dose of radiation in excess of that used in the other studies and secondly, by evaluating the use of small doses of prednisone, administered in addition to castration (see pp. 27—28). Another purpose is to see whether a measurement of endocrine function (see pp. 121—123) at the time of mastectomy can predict the response to castration.

Following mastectomy and conventional postoperative radiotherapy, the patients in MEAKIN and his colleagues' trial are being allotted by age to one of three series (Table 7). Within each series, they are then randomly assigned into treatment groups. There are two treatment groups in Series I and three treatment groups in Series II and III:

Patients aged under thirty five with tumours confined to the breast are not entered into the trial because it is not considered justifiable to castrate young women

Table 7. *Details of treatment policy in a new trial of prophylactic castration.*
(MEAKIN et al., 1968)

Series	Age of patients	Stage (TNM)	Treatment
I	35—44	2×3	NT : R
II	45—59	1,2×3	NT : R : R+P
III	60+	1,2×3	NT : R : R+P

NT   = No further treatment.
R   = Ovarian irradiation by Cobalt 60 to 2,000 rads in five days.
R+P = Ovarian irradiation as in "R", plus oral prednisone 2.5 mg three times daily.

with a good prognosis. This exclusion will negate any possible comparison with NISSEN-MEYER's premenopausal patients who, to all intents and purposes, were only those in Stage one.

Before treatment begins, each patient in Series I and II has a 24 hour urine specimen collected for hormone assays. A urine specimen is not collected from patients in Series III because the urinary hormone estimations are not reliable in patients aged over sixty.

Eventually, in each series, the treatment groups will be compared by recurrence rate, recurrence time and survival. Comparison of the results of the hormone assays with these indices of patient response may show whether assays could help in predicting those few patients on whom prophylactic ovarian ablation is really worthwhile. No results are yet available from this trial.

Surgical Castration Compared with Irradiation Castration

This is an important problem and one that the clinician has to face. Once therapeutic or prophylactic castration has been decided upon, should it be carried out by surgical removal of the ovaries or by the destruction of their function with X-irradiation? As far as the patient is concerned, there is probably little to choose between the methods. Surgical removal of the ovaries involves an abdominal operation with a general anaesthetic and so the patient must be fit enough to withstand both of these. When oophorectomy is recommended after mastectomy, the patient must be able to withstand another surgical assault (and one that is yet another attack on her femininity) after the severe emotional disturbance that may result from the primary operation. When oophorectomy is used therapeutically, it means that the patient must be physically fit enough for surgery, taking into account the extent of her metastatic disease.

Castration by irradiation also has its disadvantages. Radiotherapy is not pleasant; sickness, lethargy and depression are frequent side effects and there are many patients who would prefer a surgical operation.

If abrupt cessation of ovarian function is desired, oophorectomy must be more efficient than ovarian irradiation, and produce results more rapidly. Irradiation castration is not so certain in its effect and, in many instances, particularly in young patients, the menstrual periods have continued following treatment and on occasions even pregnancy has been reported. Presumably, the aim of ovarian ablation is to stop oestrogen secretion—at least the oestrogen which emanates from the ovaries—and therefore, some indication of the efficiency of the two methods of castration can be had from the measurement of the oestrogen excretion in the urine after treatment. BLOCK, VIAL and PULLEN (1958), using a bio-assay method for measuring oestrogens, compared the oestrogen excretion following surgical oophorectomy with that following ovarian irradiation. In a small series of eleven patients, they showed that surgical castration reduced the urinary oestrogen titre to very low levels within a period of a few days; but X-ray castration, although eventually accomplishing the same result, only did so after a long latent period. This period ranged from eighty to one hundred and thirty days. DICZFALUSY and his colleagues (1959) measured the oestrogen excretion of women at two points during their menstrual cycle and compared the levels with the excretion at two and four months after ovarian irradiation and again at two months after subsequent oophorectomy. Seventeen women were studied and the urinary excretion of oestrone, oestradiol 17β and oestriol was measured in total 96-hour urine specimens by BROWN's (1955) method. They found that ovarian irradiation significantly lowered the urinary excretion of total oestrogens and that surgical oophorectomy, performed five months later, did not further depress the level. They concluded that there was no difference in oestrogen excretion following surgical or irradiation castration. Similarly, NISSEN-MEYER and SANNER (1963) measured the excretion of oestrone, pregnanediol and pregnanetriol after castration in patients aged forty to fifty-nine years. They were unable to detect a significant difference in the urinary levels of these compounds between patients having an oophorectomy and those who had an irradiation menopause.

The best comparison of the efficiency of these treatments should be the response of the patient. When both procedures are carried out therapeutically, do patients treated by an irradiation menopause have a similar response rate to patients treated by oophorectomy? It matters little if the diminution in oestrogen excretion differs after one or other of the methods of ovarian ablation if the clinical response remains the same.

GORDON and SEGALOFF (1958) compared twenty patients, who had their ovaries removed, with twenty-nine patients who had an x-ray menopause. They reported a 40 per cent remission in the patients who had an oophorectomy compared with a 28 per cent remission in those whose ovaries were irradiated. They further observed that, if they discounted those patients in their radiation group who had their treatment carried out by the one dose technique, the remainder had a remission rate similar to those who had an oophorectomy (37 per cent). The method of treatment in these patients was not chosen by random sample.

NISSEN-MEYER (1965) carried out a clinical trial to determine which of the two methods of castration gave the better results. It may be remembered (see page 18) that his premenopausal patients with a poor prognosis were not castrated. He felt that it was unethical to include them in his trial to assess the value of ovarian ablation, because they might have been allotted to a control group and hence not treated. He did feel, however, that it was ethical to select their method of castration by random sample. 140 such patients were included in the trial, 62 receiving ovarian irradiation (by the method previously described, see page 19) and 42 having an oophorectomy. In the irradiation group, 58.2 per cent were free from disease at five years, compared with 51.3 per cent for the operation group. Similarly 71.3 per cent of patients in the irradiation group survived five years, compared with the 64.5 per cent in the operative group. The differences between the results of the two treatments were not statistically significant and NISSEN-MEYER concluded that if a difference existed, it was probably of minor importance.

The Physiological Significance of Castration

From the patient's point of view, there is little to choose between the natural menopause and an artificial menopause. In both cases, the periods stop—although perhaps more suddenly in the latter case—and in both cases the side effects may be similar; hot flushes, weight gain and psychological disturbance are just as common following ovarian ablation as after the natural menopause.

In the normal pre-menopausal woman, the ovaries secrete both oestrogen and progesterone. Oestrogens are secreted during the follicular phase and, after a brief drop at the middle of the cycle, continue to be secreted with progesterone during the luteal phase. There is still much controversy on the exact sequence of events in the normal menstrual cycle and on the relationship between pituitary F. S. H. and L. H. production and the secretion of the ovarian hormones (see BORTH, 1967).

There are now accurate chemical methods available for the measurement of the principal oestrogens excreted in the urine (BROWN, 1955; BAULD, 1956). The assay of progesterone is more difficult, but some idea of the amount secreted can be obtained by estimating the excretion of pregnanediol in the urine. Pregnanediol is a metabolic product of progesterone; it is also a metabolic product of several other substances, and hence its measurement in the urine does not give precise information on the amount of progesterone secreted.

Since oophorectomy was first used in the treatment of advanced breast cancer, it has been presumed, although with little confirmatory evidence, that the diminution or abolition of oestrogen secretion has been the principal factor in causing the cancer to regress. Following the natural menopause, oestrogen secretion certainly drops, although not to zero. The urinary excretion of pregnanediol also decreases (see for example BORTH et al., 1956, and HAYWARD et al., 1961).

An artificial menopause, whether produced by irradiation or by removal of the ovaries, seems to be similar to the natural menopause in terms of hormone excretion. After castration, oestrogen excretion diminishes and low titres are constantly observed.

NISSEN-MEYER and SANNER (1963) measured the urinary excretion of oestrone, pregnanediol and pregnanetriol in three groups of patients. One group consisted of patients who had had a natural menopause, the second group was of patients who had been castrated, and the third group was of postmenopausal patients (either spontaneous or castrated) who were also receiving prednisone 2.5 mg four times a day. Fig. 3 shows that in the first two groups the amounts of the three compounds decreased similarly with age but there was a higher excretion of oestrone in women between 50 and 60 who had had a natural menopause. In those patients receiving prednisone, the excretion of all these compounds dropped to very low levels.

It is unusual for urinary oestrogen levels to drop to zero (or at least to levels which are too low for the sensitivity of the methods of analysis) and the continued excretion probably represents oestrogens derived from adrenal secretion. The pretreatment urinary excretion of oestrogen might be expected to correlate with the response to castration or, alternatively, the response to castration might correlate in some way with the amounts of urinary oestrogen that could still be measured after treatment. Neither appears to be the case. The main difficulty in correlating pre-treatment oestrogen levels with response is that most of the patients are premenopausal. Under these circumstances, obtaining an accurate baseline measurement of oestrogen excretion would mean doing serial assays through at least one, and possible several, menstrual cycles. The work involved using the present assay methods would not make this a feasible investigation.

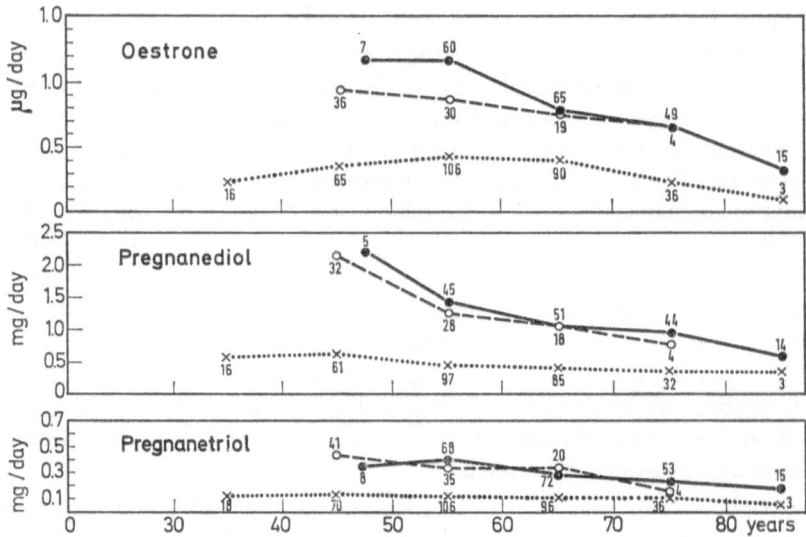

Fig. 3. Urinary excretion of oestrone, pregnanediol and pregnanetriol in **postmenopausal** women with breast cancer (NISSEN-MEYER, 1967; reproduced with permission). ●—● Spontaneous menopause; o–––o ovarian ablation; x–––x corticosteroids + ovarian ablation and/or spontaneous menopause. (Figures indicate numbers of assays in 10-years groups)

Oestrogen excretion may continue after castration and attempts have been made to correlate the levels with response. Continued oestrogen excretion has been found in successful cases and zero levels have been measured in failures. BULBROOK and his colleagues (1958) carried out a careful analysis of oestrogen excretion in patients who had had an oophorectomy. In premenopausal patients they showed that a decrease in urinary oestrogen excretion usually followed operation although there was considerable variation in the post-treatment levels. In most women, they found evidence of continued oestrogen excretion which they presumed was of adrenal origin, but they were unable to demonstrate any correlation between these levels and clinical response.

Summary and Conclusions

1. Castration is an effective therapeutic measure in many pre-menopausal patients with advanced breast cancer, although probably fewer than a third obtain benefit. It is not possible to give a true response rate because there are no agreed criteria of remission. There is no evidence on the comparative efficacy of castration and androgen administration. The successful response to therapeutic castration may herald a successful response to subsequent adrenalectomy or hypophysectomy. Occasionally, castration may be effective in postmenopausal patients but probably to a lesser degree than in premenopausal.

2. Castration performed at the time of mastectomy postpones the incidence of recurrence in pre-menopausal patients, and there may also be a favourable effect on survival. One report shows that a similar effect may be had by castrating postmenopausal patients up to the age of seventy.

3. Because prophylactic castration gives limited benefit to only a small proportion of those who are treated, it is felt that therapeutic castration may have more to offer at the present. There is a pressing need for a method of detecting those patients who will benefit

from prophylactic castration and there are trials under way at the moment to investigate this problem.

4. The results of oophorectomy do not differ significantly from the results or ovarian irradiation—providing the latter treatment is carried out using an adequate dose of x-rays. It is probably unwise to carry out ovarian irradiation by the one dose technique.

5. Urinary oestrogen and pregnanediol excretion drops after castration but small amounts of oestrogen continue to be excreted and this is probably a measure of adrenal secretion. No correlation can be found between response to castration and pre- or post-operative levels of urinary oestrogen.

References

ADAIR, F. E., TREVES, N., FARROW, J. H., SCHARNAGEL, I. M.: Clinical effects of surgical and x-ray castration in mammary cancer. J. Amer. med. Ass. 128, 161 (1945).

ALRICH, E. M., LIDDLE, H. V., MORTON, C. B., II.: Carcinoma of the breast. Results of surgical treatment. Some anatomic and endocrine considerations. Ann. Surg. 145, 799 (1957).

BAULD, W. S.: A method for the determination of Oestriol, Oestrone and Oestradiol-17β in human urine by partition chromatography and colorimetric estimation. Biochem. J. 63, 488 (1956).

BEATSON, G. W.: On the treatment of inoperable cases of carcinoma of the mamma: suggestions for a new method of treatment with illustrative cases. Lancet 1896 II, 104, 162.

BLOCK, G. E., VIAL, A. B., PULLEN, F. W.: Oestrogen excretion following operative and irradiation castration in cases of mammary cancer. Surgery 43, 415 (1958).

BORTH, R.: Endocrinology of the human menstrual cycle: opinions and hypotheses. Vitam. and Horm. 25, 123 (1967).

— LINDER, A., RIONDEL, A.: Urinary excretion of 17-hydroxy-corticosteroids and 17-keto-steroids in healthy subjects in relation to sex, age, body weight and height. Acta endocr. (Kbh.) 25, 33 (1957).

BOYD, S.: On Oophorectomy in cancer of the breast. Brit. med. J. 1900 II, 1161.

BROWN, J. B.: A chemical method for the determination of Oestriol, Oestrone and Oestradiol in the human urine. Biochem. J. 60, 185 (1955).

BULBROOK, R. D., GREENWOOD, F. C., HADFIELD, G. J., SCOWEN, E. F.: Oophorectomy in breast cancer. An attempt to correlate clinical results with oestrogen production. Brit. med. J. 1958 II, 7.

COLE, MARY P.: The place of radiotherapy in the management of early breast cancer. Brit. J. Surg. 51, 216 (1964).

COLE, M. P.: Suppression of ovarian function in primary breast cancer. In: Prognostic Factors in Breast Cancer. Eds.: A. P. M. FORREST and P. B. KUNKLER. Edinburgh: Livingstone 1968, p. 146.

Co-operative Breast Cancer Group. Protocol 1 — A co-operative study to evaluate experimental steroids in the therapy of advanced carcinoma. In: Clinical Evaluation in Breast Cancer. Eds.: J. L. HAYWARD and R. D. BULBROOK. London-New York: Academic Press 1966, p. 275.

DAO, T. L., NEMOTO, T.: An evaluation of adrenalectomy and androgen in disseminated mammary carcinoma. Surg. Gynec. Obstet. 121, 1257 (1965).

— — BROSS, I.: A controlled randomised comparative study of early and late adrenalectomy in women with advanced breast cancer. In Prognostic Factors in Breast Cancer. Eds.: A. P. M. FORREST and P. B. KUNKLER. Edinburgh: Livingstone 1968, p. 177.

DICZFALUSY, E., NOTTER, G., EDSMYR, F., WESTMAN, A.: Oestrogen excretion in breast cancer patients before and after ovarian irradiation and oophorectomy. J. clin. Endocr. 19, 1230 (1959).

DOUGLAS, M.: The treatment of advanced breast cancer by hormone therapy. Brit. J. Cancer 6, 32 (1952).

EMERSON, K. J., JR., JESSIMAN, H. G.: Hormonal influences on growth and progression of cancer: tests for hormone dependency in mammary and prostatic cancer. New Engl. J. Med. 254, 252 (1956).

FAIRGRIEVE, J.: Selective criteria for surgical removal of the endocrine glands. Surg. Gynec. Obstet. 120, 371 (1965).

FRACCHIA, A. A., FARROW, J. H., DE PALO, A. J., CONNOLLY, D. P., HUVOS, A. G.: Castration for primary inoperable or recurrent breast carcinoma. Surg. Gynec. Obstet. 128, 1226 (1969).

GORDON, D. L., SEGALOFF, A.: Castration as a palliative therapy for advanced breast cancer. The Second Biennial Louisiana Cancer Conference. Ed.: A. SEGALOFF. St. Louis: C. V. Mosby Co. 1958, p. 187.

HALL, T. C., DEDERICK, M. M., NEVINNY, H. B., MUENCH, H.: Prognostic value of response of patients with breast cancer to therapeutic castration. Cancer Chemother. Rep. 31, 47 (1963).

HAYWARD, J. L., BULBROOK, R. D. (eds.): Clinical Evaluation in Breast Cancer. London-New York: Academic Press 1966.

— — Urinary steroids and prognosis in breast cancer. In: Prognostic Factors in Breast Cancer. Eds.: A. P. M. FORREST and P. B. KUNKLER. Edinburgh: Livingstone 1968, p. 383.

— — GREENWOOD, F. C.: Hormone assays and prognosis in breast cancer. Mem. Soc. Endocr. 10, 144 (1961).

HERMAN, G. E.: Four cases of recurrent mammary carcinoma treated by oophorectomy and thyroid extract. Brit. med. J. 1900 II, 1167.

HUCK, P.: Artificial menopause as an adjunct to radical treatment of breast cancer. N. Z. med. J. 51, 364 (1952).

KENNEDY, B. J.: The role of castration in breast cancer. Surgery 88, 743 (1964).

— FORTUNY, I. E.: Therapeutic castration in the treatment of advanced breast cancer. Cancer 17, 1197 (1964).

— MIELKE, P. W., FORTUNY, I. E.: Therapeutic castration versus prophylactic castration in breast cancer. Surg. Gynec. Obstet. 118, 524 (1964).

LEMON, H. M.: Cortisone-thyroid therapy of metastatic breast cancer. Ann. intern. Med. 46, 457 (1957).

— Prednisone therapy of advanced mammary cancer. Cancer 12, 93 (1959).

LEWISON, E. F.: Prophylactic versus therapeutic castration in the total treatment of breast cancer. Obstet. gynec. Surv. 17, 769 (1962).

— Castration in the treatment of advanced breast cancer. Cancer 18, 1558 (1965).

LOESER, A. A.: A new therapy for prevention of postoperative recurrences in genital and breast cancer. Brit. med. J. 1954 II, 1380.

MACDONALD, I.: The role of extirpative procedures in cancer of the breast. Cancer 10, 805 (1957).

McWHIRTER, R.: Some factors influencing prognosis in breast cancer. J. Fac. Radiol. (Lond.) 8, 220 (1956).

MEAKIN, J. W., ALLT, W. E. C., BEALE, F. A., BROWN, T. C., CLARK, K. M., FITZPATRICK, P. F., HAWKINS, N. V., JENKIN, R. D. T., BULBROOK, R. D., HAYWARD, J. L.: A preliminary report of two studies of adjuvant treatment of primary breast cancer. In: Prognostic Factors in Breast Cancer. Eds.: A. P. M. FORREST and P. B. KUNKLER. Edinburgh: Livingstone 1968, p. 157.

MOORE, F. D., WOODROW, S. I., ALIAPOULIOS, M. A., WILSON, R. E.: Carcinoma of the Breast. Boston: Little, Brown 1968, p. 45.

MYERS, W. P. L., WEST, C. D., PEARSON, O. H., KARNOTSKY, D. A.: Androgen-induced exacerbation of breast cancer measured by calcium excretion: conversion of androgen to estrogen as possible underlying mechanism. J. Amer. med. Ass. 161, 127 (1956).

NISSEN-MEYER, R.: Castration as part of the primary treatment for operable female breast cancer. Acta radiol. (Stockh.) Suppl. 249 (1965).

— The role of prophylactic castration in the therapy of human mammary cancer. Europ. J. Cancer. 3, 395 (1967).

— SANNER, T.: The excretion of oestrone, pregnandiol and pregnanetriol in breast cancer patients. II effect of ovariectomy, ovarian irradiation and corticosteroids. Acta endocr. (Kbh.) 44, 334 (1963).

NOVAK, E. R., WILLIAMS, T. J.: Autopsy comparison of cardiovascular changes in the castrated and normal woman. Amer. J. Obstet. Gynec. 80, 863 (1960).

Oliver, M. F., Boyd, G. S.: Effect of bilateral oophorectomy on coronary-artery disease and serum lipid levels. Lancet 1959 II, 691.

Peters, M. Vera: The effect of pregnancy in breast cancer. In: Prognostic Factors in Breast Cancer. Eds.: A. P. M. Forrest and P. B. Kunkler. Edinburgh: Livingstone 1968, p. 65.

Rennaes, S.: Cancer of the breast in women, a clinical and statistical investigation of the material of the Norwegian Radium Hospital 1932—51. Acta chir. scand. Suppl. 266, 85 (1960).

Rosenberg, M. F., Uhlmann, E. M.: Prophylactic castration in carcinoma of the breast. Arch. Surg. 78, 376 (1959).

Smith, G. U., Smith, O. W.: Carcinoma of the breast, results, evaluation of x-irradiation, and relation of age and surgical castration to length of survival. Surg. Gynec. Obstet. 97, 508 (1953).

Smithers, D. W.: Cancer of the breast and the menopause. J. Fac. Radiol. (Lond.) 4, 89 (1952—53).

Sznajderman, M., Oliver, M. F.: Spontaneous premature menopause, ischemic heart disease, and serum lipids. Lancet 1963 I, 962.

Taylor, G. W.: Evaluation of ovarian sterilization for breast cancer. Surg. Gynec. Obstet. 68, 452 (1939).

Taylor, S. G., III: Endocrine ablation in disseminated mammary carcinoma. Surg. Gynec. Obstet. 115, 443 (1962).

Treves, N.: An evaluation of prophylactic castration in the treatment of mammary carcinoma. Cancer 10, 393 (1957).

— Finkbeiner, J. A.: An evaluation of therapeutic surgical castration in the treatment of metastatic, recurrent, and primary inoperable mammary carcinoma in women. Cancer 11, 421 (1958).

Wagoner, J. K., Chiazze, L., Jr., William Lloyd, I.: Cancer of the breast at menopausal ages. Cancer 20, 354 (1967).

Wilson, R. E., Jessiman, A. G., Moore, F. D.: Severe exacerbation of cancer of the breast after oophorectomy and adrenalectomy. New Engl. J. Med. 258, 312 (1958).

Chapter 3

The Adrenals and the Pituitary

It is now over fifteen years since adrenalectomy and hypophysectomy were first successfully performed to treat advanced breast cancer. The rationale for their use had been appreciated for many years but previous attempts to carry out the operations had been thwarted by lack of suitable replacement therapy. HUGGINS in Chicago had carried out an adrenalectomy in 1945 (HUGGINS and DAO, 1953) and ATKINS had performed several partial adrenalectomies for breast cancer by 1947 (ATKINS, 1966 b). Removal of the normal pituitary gland had been achieved even earlier—CHABANNIER had carried out a hypophysectomy for diabetes mellitus by 1936 (CHABANNIER et al., 1936)—but these attempts were similarly frustrated by lack of effective replacement therapy. Then, in the early fifties, cortisone was synthesised and, for the first time, the adrenal and pituitary glands could be removed with safety. The late effects of removal of these glands were then unknown and it was not unnatural that surgeons should think that a panacea was now available for many ailments that previously had been untreatable. Diabetes, exophthalmic goitre, Cushings disease, hypertension and cancer were all at one time or another treated by adrenalectomy or hypophysectomy. Eventually, in each of these conditions, due appraisal was made of the effect of the operations and in most cases they were abandoned. Nowadays, with few exceptions, the normal pituitary or adrenal glands are removed only in cases of breast or prostatic carcinoma, Cushing's disease or for diabetic retinopathy.

The operations have been carried out on innumerable occasions. Reports of five hundred (FRACCHIA et al., 1967) or even a thousand (PROHASKA, 1967) adrenalectomies are now in the literature, and large series of hypophysectomies have also been reported (see for instance LUFT et al., 1958; RAY and PEARSON, 1958; PEARSON and RAY, 1960; KENNEDY and FRENCH, 1965). The results of both operations have been completely reviewed and assessed (see DAO, 1960; CUTLER, 1962). But the results are variable (GORDAN, 1967) and there is still no clear indication of exactly what are the chances of a favourable response and what this favourable response will achieve in terms of remission and longevity.

Nevertheless, many prospective and retrospective investigations have been planned, analysed and reported. Individually the results of such investigations may not have contributed a great deal, but taken together they have furthered our understanding of the indications for endocrine ablation and the mechanism of response.

1. The Remission Rates from Adrenalectomy and Hypophysectomy

The assessment of response to adrenalectomy or hypophysectomy does not present all the difficulties that were encountered when assessing the response to castration. This is probably because the treatment is more severe and hence there is a greater need for a proper understanding of what can be achieved. More purposeful work has been done and, in its analysis, greater attention has been paid to selecting suitable criteria for judging response. Whilst no agreement has been reached on exactly what should be accepted as an objective remission, possible by chance, many workers have happened to select almost identical criteria of success.

It has been suggested firstly, that only objective response shall be accepted as evidence of remission; secondly, that most or all lesions must improve without any new lesions occurring; and thirdly, that this remission must have a minimum time limit. Six months is usually proposed (see for instance PROHASKA, 1967; HAYWARD, 1966; MACDONALD, 1962). Under these circumstances, there is a remarkable agreement on the response rate. Whether it is an adrenalectomy or a hypophysectomy that has been carried out, approximately 30 per cent of the patients will obtain a remission. By definition, this remission must last at least six months, but reports of a duration of six to eight years are not uncommon.

Thus, provided the operations are carried out skilfully, a surgeon can confidently expect that about one patient in three will derive worthwhile benefit. One of the first problems that necessitated more specific enquiry was the question whether adrenalectomy gave the same degree of benefit as hypophysectomy.

PEARSON and RAY (1959) compared 67 of their patients who had had an adrenalectomy with 89 who had had a hypophysectomy. They concluded that hypophysectomy appeared to be superior to adrenalectomy in both remission rate and survival although the differences were not significant. However, they pointed out that their comparison was fraught with difficulties because the procedures were carried out at different times (adrenalectomy, 1951—1955, hypophysectomy, 1954—1956) and no attempt was made at pairing or randomisation.

Two investigations have been undertaken to compare adrenalectomy with hypophysectomy and each has been reported twice. One investigation was by retrospective enquiry (Joint Committee on Endocrine Ablative Procedures in Disseminated Mammary Carcinoma, 1961, MACDONALD, 1962) and the other by a prospective clinical trial (ATKINS et al., 1957 and 1960). Eventually, the two investigations drew different conclusions and, because two fundamentally different types of clinical enquiry were used, it is important to know the reason for disagreement.

(i) The Joint Committee investigated the results of the operations of adrenalectomy and hypophysectomy in twelve different medical centres. The analysis was done by an internist who reviewed the medical records, abstracted the details of the patients' history and treatment and decided by retrospective review whether each patient had had an objective response. Patients who had died within one month of operation or who had had only a local recurrence of their disease after mastectomy were not included. Other patients were excluded because the follow-up was not long enough. In its first report (1961) the Joint Committee gave the response rate following adrenalectomy as being 31.7 per cent and the response rate after hypophysectomy as 31.3 per cent. The mean survival of the successful adrenalectomy patients was

22.0 months and of the successful hypophysectomies, 20.6 months. The mean survival of unresponsive patients was also similar, 7.0 months and 6.5 months respectively.

The final report of this investigations was published a year later (MACDONALD, 1962). Here, nearly double the number of adrenalectomies (690 compared with 367) and slightly fewer hypophysectomies (340 compared with 358 were similarly analysed. The response rate from adrenalectomy was now reported as 28.4 per cent and the response rate from hypophysectomy as 32.6 per cent. The survival from ablation to death for responsive and unresponsive patients was similar to that given in the first report. MACDONALD concluded that there was no significant difference between the effectiveness of adrenalectomy and hypophysectomy.

(ii) ATKINS and his colleagues investigated the same problem by means of a controlled clinical trial. Patients with advanced breast cancer were accepted into this trial only after preliminary hormone therapy (androgens in premenopausal women and oestrogens in postmenopausal women) had been tried and failed. The patients were then independently examined by a physician to assess their fitness both for adrenalectomy and hypophysectomy. Only if they were fit enough for either procedure were they entered into the trial. They were allocated by random sample (a ticket was drawn from a box) either to adrenalectomy with oophorectomy or to hypophysectomy. Adrenalectomy was carried out in two stages: at the first stage, the right adrenal and both ovaries were removed and at the second stage, about ten days later, the left adrenal was removed. Hypophysectomy was carried out by the transfrontal route.

The patients were followed up at monthly intervals until death. At each follow-up visit, a comparison was made with the clinical condition before treatment. The effectiveness of the operations was compared by the Mean Clinical Value (M.C.V.) or the Survival Rate. The M.C.V. has been described in detail elsewhere (HAYWARD, 1966), but can be summarised as follows.

Before treatment, all lesions are measured and the measurements are recorded on a card. The lesions are allotted to systems; for instances, all involved lymph nodes would be entered as lymphatic system, skin nodules as cutaneous system, etc. At four weekly intervals, the same lesions are measured and the measurements are compared with those recorded before treatment. If a lesion has got smaller, it is given 2 marks, if it is the same size, it is given 1 mark and if it is bigger, it is given 0. To give a score for the system, these marks are then averaged and multiplied by 6 to bring to a convenient number. The score for the patient as a whole is obtained by averaging the system marks. Thus, if all lesions have improved, the M.C.V. will be 12, if all lesions have deteriorated, the M.C.V. will be 0 and a figure between 0 and 12 will indicate gradations of response. The monthly M.C.V.'s are plotted on a chart and the progress of a patient can be seen at a glance. Figure 4 shows the working of the M.C.V. for one system, and Figure 5, a typical M.C.V. chart. Comparisons of groups of patients can be made by using both the average M.C.V. for the group at three months and the average area under the M.C.V. curve—the latter figure giving a measure of length of survival as well as of remission. It is an accurate system and is particularly valuable in the statistical comparison of the response to treatment of groups of patients.

In their first report, ATKINS and his colleagues (1957) were able to compare the response of thirty patients after adrenalectomy with thirty patients after hypophys-

Before treatment

> For M.C.V.

> System 1: Lymphatic

> 1. Left axilla node $\frac{1}{2}'' \times \frac{3}{8}''$
> 2. Right supraclavicular fossa node $\frac{1}{2}''$ diam.
> 3. Left supraclavicular fossa node $\frac{1}{4}''$ diam.

At first visit after treatment

> System 1: Lymphatic

> 1. Left axilla node $\frac{1}{4}'' \times \frac{3}{8}''$ —improved (2)
> 2. Right supraclavicular fossa node $\frac{1}{2}''$ diam.—same (1)
> 3. Left supraclavicular fossa node impalpable—improved (2)

$$\text{M.C.V.} = \frac{\text{total marks}}{\text{number of lesions}} = \text{average mark} \times 6 \text{ (to bring to suitable number)}$$

$$= \frac{2+1+2}{3} \times 6 = 10$$

Fig. 4. The calculation of the "Mean Clinical Value"

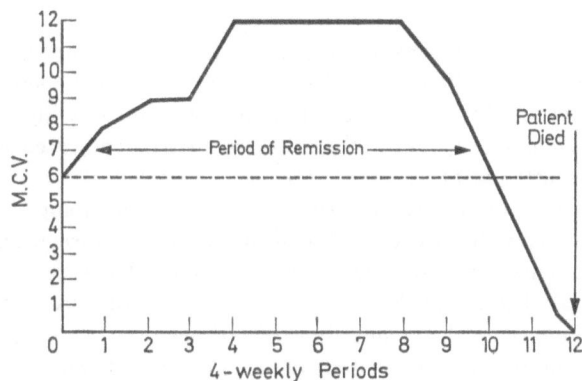

Fig. 5. Typical M.C.V. chart of a patient who obtained ten months response following adrenalectomy

ectomy. Both the degree of remission (as measured by the M.C.V.) and the survival rate were better for the hypophysectomy patients but the differences were not significant. In their second report (ATKINS et al., 1960), ATKINS' group compared the response of seventy nine adrenalectomy patients with the response of seventy hypophysectomy patients. The trend observed in the earlier report continued; hypophysectomy gave superior results, both in remission and survival, but this time the differences were significant in both the M.C.V. at three months and in the proportional survival of the two groups (see Table 8). The extent of the difference was still not great and, although achieving formal statistical significance, it was not felt to be sufficiently large to dictate treatment policy.

Table 8. *Comparison of the results of adrenalectomy and hypophysectomy in a randomised trial.* (Atkins et al., 1960)

	Adrenalectomy		Hypophysectomy		Difference between means ± standard error	S.E. diff. (t)
	No. of patients	Mean value	No. of patients	Mean value		
Mean clinical value						
At 3 months	79	5.16	70	6.95	1.79 ±0.76	2.35 ⊥
At 6 months	72	4.52	66	6.18	1.66 ±0.87	1.89
At 1 year	70[a]	2.91	61[a]	4.34	1.43 ±0.85	1.68
Log (total M.C.V.)	79	1.548	70	1.769	0.221 ±0.098	2.26‡
Average M.C.V.	79	5.48	70	6.57	1.09 ±0.48	2.28‡
Survival (by life-table)						
Proportion surviving						
At 3 months	—	0.666	—	0.812	0.146±0.071	2.05⁸
At 6 months	—	0.596	—	0.678	0.082±0.080	1.02
At 1 year	—	0.405	—	0.567	0.162±0.084	1.92
Expectation of life (months)	—	14.2	—	20.3	6.1 ±3.6	1.70

[a] Nine patients in each category were followed up for less than a year. Significance of differences: ⊥ 0.01 < P < 0.02 ‡ 0.02 < P < 0.03 ⁸ 0.04 < P < 0.05

These two enquiries, each measuring the response of patients to adrenalectomy or hypophysectomy, gave different results. The retrospective review indicated that there was no significant difference in the response of patients with advanced breast cancer to the two operations, whilst the randomised trial indicated that hypophysectomy was significantly better.

Both enquiries have been criticised. In the review by the Joint Committee, there were many gaps in the published data. For instance, little information was given on the number of patients that, for various reasons, must have been considered and rejected for the trial. There must have been a high degree of selection and this could have had a major effect on the results; it is disturbing that fewer hypophysectomies were analysed in the second report than in the first. No details were given of the operative technique and, possibly more important, on how many of the hypophysectomies were carried out by surgeons who perform the operation only occasionally. When infrequently performed, hypophysectomy can be an operation with a high morbidity rate, also significant amounts of viable pituitary tissue may be left in the pituitary fossa in a large proportion of cases.

On the other hand, the randomised trial carried out by Atkins and his colleagues did no more than report the results under a particularly narrow set of circumstances —the operations were carried out by particular surgeons in a particular manner and always in the same hospital. Except under these stringent conditions, it did not provide an answer to the question which of the two operations gives better results in the treatment of advanced breast cancer. There is perhaps some scientific interest in the marginal advantage in survival and remission induced by hypophysectomy— a finding common to Atkins' trial, the Joint Committee's review and also the investigation by Pearson and Ray (1959)—but it would only need a slight rise in morbidity, or the occasional operation to be incomplete, and the advantage that hypophysectomy holds over adrenalectomy would be reversed. Adrenalectomy can be carried out by any competent general surgeon and must still be considered the operation of choice when ablative procedures are only occasionally undertaken.

The comparison between the two trials is interesting in the light of present day thinking on clinical experimentation. The randomised investigation reported by the ATKINS group was one of the first controlled clinical trials on cancer reported in the medical literature. The properly controlled randomised study should give a complete and accurate answer to the question which of two treatments gives better results, but ATKINS and his colleagues' trial was too narrow in it's concept. Although randomisation infered that the two groups were comparable and that no selection had taken place, their treatment was not representative of what is available in ordinary surgical practice. ATKINS (1966 a) himself has since commented that the whole investigation had such a local and restricted significance that the differences were not generally meaningful.

The investigation by the Joint Committee pointed out the pitfalls of a trial by retrospective enquiry. As CUTLER (1966) has pointed out, retrospective review has a place as a method of giving a lead for further study. But probably it should not be used to compare two methods of treatment. STRONG (1963) even remarked that "... This conclusion (that adrenalectomy and hypophysectomy gave equivalent results), based as it is on nearly 1,200 patients, is perhaps an indictment of clinical investigation by committee ..."

Perhaps these two studies should be regarded as evolutionary phases in the development of methods for clinical enquiry. Neither produced results which have been of practical clinical use but, by example, each may have helped in the design of future clinical experiments.

2. The Timing of Adrenalectomy and Hypophysectomy

Because adrenalectomy and hypophysectomy are major operations and because they are only palliative in their effect, their use is usually reserved for patients on whom all other forms of treatment have failed. A cure is never possible nor do the operations help all the patients on whom they are performed; at the best about one third of those who are treated gain a few years of relatively normal symptom-free life. The common practice is first to try the effect of local surgery, radiotherapy, hormone therapy and sometimes cytotoxins and only to recommend a major ablative procedure when these measures have failed. This policy was particularly popular when the operations were still in the experimental stage. In the early 1950's, it was believed that these largely untried major procedures should be performed only on patients with very advanced disease but it was also appreciated that such a conservative policy might well negate much of the benefit that might be obtained from the operations. It was optimistic to expect an operation to succeed when it was only attempted as a last resort and possibly the rewards would be greater if the operation was performed earlier, when recurrences and metastases were only beginning to appear. There were many precedents for this in surgical history—for example, mitral valvotomy might well have been discarded as a treatment for mitral stenosis in the light of some of the poor early results when the operation was performed only on grossly incapacitated patients.

The general experience seemed to be that only about two thirds of those patients presenting with advanced breast cancer, and on whom hormone therapy or castration had been tried, survived to have an adrenalectomy or hypophysectomy. The problem was to determine whether a greater degree of palliation and longer survival would result from operating earlier without using hormone therapy or castration as a preliminary measure.

This question was investigated in a prospective trial (ATKINS et al., 1966; HAYWARD, 1967). 191 patients with advanced breast cancer, who had had no previous endocrine therapy, were included. They were passed as fit both for hormone therapy and endocrine ablation before they were considered. Then, either they were treated immediately by adrenalectomy or hypophysectomy and without previous hormone therapy (operation group) or they were treated by hormones first and an adrenalectomy or hypophysectomy only carried out when the hormone therapy had failed (conservative group). The allocation of each patient to one or other of the treatment groups was made by random sample.

The results of therapy in the two groups were compared by three methods:

1. Survival experience.
2. The degree and duration of remission as expressed by the M. C. V. (see pp. 34—35).
3. The success rates from hormone therapy and ablation.

1. The survival experience of the two groups was remarkably similar. Figure 6 shows the survival curves for the operation and control groups, calculated on the life table principle. Table 9 gives data which have been extracted from the life table, indicating the similar proportions in each group, surviving to three, six and twelve months; the calculated expectation of life differs by only 0.1 months.

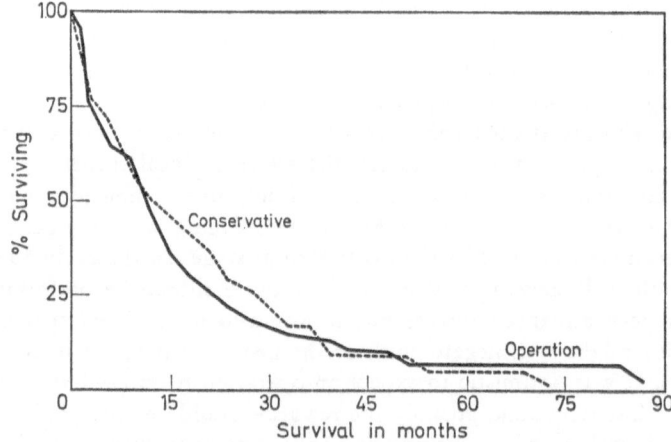

Fig. 6. Life table showing the survival experience of the "operation" and "conservative" groups. (ATKINS et al., 1966)

Table 9. *The "operation" and "conservative" groups compared by survival proportions and expectation, calculated from the life table shown in Figure 6.* (ATKINS et al., 1966)

Survival from life table	Operation group	Conservative group
Proportions surviving to:		
3 months	0.766	0.783
6 months	0.649	0.701
12 months	0.478	0.515
Calculated expectation of life	17.9 months	17.8 months

Table 10. *The remission experience of the "operation" and "conservative" groups.* (ATKINS et al., 1966)

	Operation group	Conservative group
Mean survival	14.94 months	15.46 months
Mean period of remission	8.98 months	7.65 months
Per cent of survival spent in remission	60.0%	49.0%

Table 11. *The results of hormone therapy in the "conservative" group and of operation in both groups.* (ATKINS et al., 1966)

	Operation group	Conservative group
Results from hormones		
Success		15 (16%)
Intermediate	—	20 (21%)
Failure		60 (63%)
Results from endocrine ablation		
Success	28 (30%)	13 (23%)
Intermediate	17 (18%)	16 (28%)
Failure	49 (52%)	28 (49%)

2. Table 10 indicates the mean period of remission experienced by patients in the two groups. Again, the results are very similar although a greater percentage of survival is spent in remission in the operation group than in the conservative group.

3. Table 11 shows the results of hormone therapy in the conservative group and the results of operation in both groups, expressed in terms of the success rate (see HAYWARD, 1966). This table shows that the success rate following ablation is lower if previous hormone therapy has been given, than if the operations are carried out *de novo;* also, that of the ninety seven patients allocated to the conservative group only fifty seven (61 per cent) survived to have a subsequent adrenalectomy or hypophysectomy.

Nevertheless, the expectation of survival was almost identical in the two groups and the small differences observed in the period of remission were not significant.

In the light of these results, it was felt that the decision whether to give hormones first or to recommend an immediate adrenalectomy or hypophysectomy need not be influenced by the expectation of an appreciable difference in survival or remission, although there was evidence that previous hormone therapy decreased the likelihood of response to subsequent ablation. Conventional methods of treatment (hormone therapy, etc. first, followed later by an ablative procedure) seemed to be to the greatest advantage of the patient.

A trial along similar lines was carried out by DAO and NEMOTO (1965). Essentially, they were comparing adrenalectomy with androgen therapy but some of their results have a bearing on the timing of ablative procedures. They divided their patients into three groups: the patients in one group undergoing immediate adrenalectomy, in another receiving one of two standard androgen preparations and in a third having an androgen compound of unknown potency. The allocation of patients to the three groups was made by random sample. To assess response, DAO and NEMOTO used the protocol of the Co-operative Breast Cancer Group (SEGALOFF, 1966) which is similar to that described on page 33 except that no minimum time limit is set in the definition of success. They noted a 45 per cent (39/86) success rate from adrenalectomy but only a 16 per cent (11/67) success rate following administration of one of the reference androgen compounds (only two out of eighty eight patients had a successful response to the test androgens). Seventy five, of the 175 patients receiving androgen therapy, went on to ablation, and the 35 per cent remission rate of these patients was less (but not significantly so) than the 45 per cent remission rate of those undergoing adrenalectomy as a primary measure. No attempt was made to assess the survival or remission experience enjoyed by the patients throughout all treatments.

In a subsequent report, including more patients (DAO et al., 1968), the survival of patients treated by immediate adrenalectomy was found to be longer than the survival of those treated initially by androgen therapy, but the difference was not significant. Also the subsequent success rate from adrenalectomy, in those patients first receiving standard androgen preparations (response rate 16 per cent), was 28 per cent, whereas the success rate from adrenalectomy in those patients receiving the experimental compounds (response rate 2.9 per cent) was 40 per cent. This seems to indicate that a remission from androgen therapy may be obtained at the expense of a subsequent remission from adrenalectomy.

FORREST et al. (1968), have also described the preliminary results of a trial they are undertaking to investigate the timing of pituitary ablation. They are comparing the remission rate of patients undergoing immediate ablation by 90 Yttrium implant with the remission rate of another group of patients—matched and randomised in pairs—in which no immediate implant is being performed. They state that their preliminary results on 119 patients agree with those of ATKINS et al. (1966) and suggest that in terms of survival, there is nothing to be gained by early endocrine ablation.

Another similar trial has been reported by SELLWOOD et al. (1968). Here, patients in one group are being treated by immediate pituitary ablation using 90 Yttrium whilst those in the other group are having a pituitary ablation only after a trial of hormone therapy—fluoxymesterone in premenopausal women, and stilboestrol followed by fluoxymesterone in postmenopausal women. A preliminary analysis of 100 patients has shown no marked difference in remission or survival between the two groups.

Another aspect of this problem is the question whether anything would be gained by carrying out ablation at a much earlier stage in the disease—indeed, before secondaries have developed. Adrenalectomy or hypophysectomy might be recommended as a "prophylactic" measure after mastectomy, in the same way as castration is sometimes used (see pp 15—19). Suitable patients might be those found at mastectomy to have a particularly virulent type of tumour, typified by a histological grade indicating high malignancy, and also presenting with gross involvement of the axillary glands. DRAGSTEDT et al. (1960) described a patient who had had a bilateral adrenalectomy and oophorectomy carried out as a prophylactic measure. The patient was a twenty-seven year old girl with an infiltrating tumour of the breast and considerable lymphatic involvement. Bilateral adrenalectomy was carried out eight months after mastectomy, when she was still without evidence of recurrence or metastases. She was still alive and free from overt disease ten years later (DRAGSTEDT, 1961). PATEY (1960) described eleven patients who had had an adrenalectomy with oophorectomy performed as a prophylactic measure. Patients were selected whose prognosis was considered bad (principally those who were shown to have metastatic growth in both the axillary and internal mammary nodes) and the adrenalectomy was carried out within a few months of mastectomy. In fact, by the time adrenalectomy was performed, five of the original eleven patients already had evidence of recurrence although this was localised and only minor in extent. At the time of PATEY's report, six of the eleven patients had died of recurrence and in another the disease had recurred but she was still alive. Of the four who were alive and free from disease, the longest survivor was still within four years of adrenalectomy. PATEY concluded from his preliminary results that adrenalectomy was unlikely to offer a significant contribution to the treatment of early carcinoma of the breast.

3. The Comparative Results of Hormone Therapy and Ablation

Some aspects of the comparative effects of hormone therapy and ablation have been discussed in the previous section on the timing of adrenalectomy and hypophysectomy. In the trials, comparing the effects of early and late endocrine ablation, some information was gathered on the relative merits of endocrine ablation and hormone therapy.

The trial reported by DAO and NEMOTO (1965) compared directly, in postmenopausal women, the response rate following androgen administration with the response rate following bilateral adrenalectomy. In their more recent report (DAO et al., 1968), they showed that fifty out of 108 patients (45 per cent) had an objective remission following adrenalectomy, compared with seventeen out of 106 patients (16 per cent) who had a remission following androgen therapy.

ATKINS et al. (1966) were able to compare the response rate of ninety four patients, randomised for adrenalectomy or hypophysectomy, with the response rate of ninety seven patients, randomised for hormone therapy. These patients were both pre- and postmenopausal, the premenopausal were given androgen therapy and the postmenopausal oestrogen therapy. Table 11 shows the response rate from the two methods of treatment. Thirty per cent of those recommended for ablation had a successful response, compared with 16 per cent of those recommended for hormone therapy. Thus adrenalectomy or hypophysectomy gave approximately twice the remission rate obtained from hormone therapy. DAO and his colleagues' (1968) series showed adrenalectomy to give three times the remission rate obtained from androgen therapy. This difference between the series reported by ATKINS et al. (1966) and by DAO et al. (1968) may be accounted for by the different techniques of hormone administration. The remission rate from endocrine ablation reported by ATKINS and his colleagues was also low (30 per cent), probably because their criteria of remission were slightly stricter than those used by DAO et al. BYRON (1967) has also compared bilateral adrenalectomy with hormone therapy in randomised series. The hormones used were either androgens, oestrogens or corticosteroids, although it is not clear what were the indications for each. Although BYRON did not detail his criteria of response, he gave his objective remission rate from adrenalectomy as 31 per cent (13/42 patients) and his remission rate from hormone therapy as 22 per cent (9/40 patients). BYRON also commented that he found the side effects from adrenalectomy minor compared with the effects of hormone therapy.

These three series report that endocrine ablation gives a better remission rate than hormone therapy by half as much again (BYRON, 1967), twice as much (ATKINS et al., 1966) and three times as much (DAO et al., 1968). The only constant finding is that ablation is superior. The series all differ from one another in their concept of what is meant by hormone therapy and this could easily account for the variations in remission rate. What is shown by these three series is the danger of relying on the result of one trial, however well randomised and well controlled; only minor changes in protocol can give major alterations in results.

Other investigations into the comparative effects of ablation and hormone therapy have concerned the use of corticosteroids. Corticosteroids have been used for many years to treat advanced breast cancer and it is believed that they may act in a different way from androgens or oestrogens. The term "medical adrenalectomy" has been used to describe their mode of action in the belief that they have a similar physiological effect as bilateral surgical adrenalectomy. If this is so, the response rate following their administration should mimic very closely that observed following adrenalectomy. If the results from corticosteroids were very similar to those from adrenalectomy and possibly hypophysectomy, the need for the operations would disappear.

DAO, TAN and BROOKES (1961) have published the results of a trial comparing adrenalectomy with cortisone therapy in the treatment of advanced breast cancer. The trial included thirty-nine patients, all of whom were postmenopausal and had previously been treated with androgens or oestrogens. They were allocated by random sample to two groups; the nineteen patients in one group had a bilateral adrenalectomy and the twenty patients in the other group were given cortisone therapy and only referred for adrenalectomy if their disease failed to respond to cortisone. Of the eighteen adrenalectomy patients who could be assessed, eight (44.5 per cent) had an objective response, whereas none of the nineteen patients receiving cortisone obtained any benefit from the treatment. Subsequently, seven of the patients who failed to respond to cortisone therapy had an adrenalectomy from which two had a remission. DAO and his colleagues concluded that these results stress the worthwhile value of adrenalectomy and demonstrate that the benefit obtained from the operation is not attributable to the steroid replacement therapy.

This trial was designed not to compare the results from corticosteroid therapy with those from adrenalectomy, but rather to investigate whether the response after adrenalectomy was due to the replacement therapy. The prescription of corticosteroids (usually prednisone is prescribed) can be an effective treatment for patients with advanced breast cancer (see Chapter 6), but probably bigger doses of steroids are needed than were used in the trial described by DAO et al. (1961).

FORREST et al. (1968) have more recently described a study in which steroid therapy plus oophorectomy is being compared with surgical adrenalectomy. Preliminary reports on sixty three patients who have been included in the trial indicate that the suppression of adrenal function by steroid administration is not as effective as surgical ablation.

4. Techniques

a) Adrenalectomy

The term "total adrenalectomy" usually infers that not only are both adrenals removed, but also both ovaries. Exceptions will be in those cases where the ovaries have been removed previously, either as a prophylactic measure following mastectomy or as treatment for the advanced disease. Essentially, adrenalectomy can be performed by one of two techniques. Either both adrenals may be removed in one operation, through an upper abdominal incision, or the operation may be done in two stages. At the first stage, the right adrenal is removed through an incision in the right flank and thence via the bed of the eleventh or twelfth rib; at the second stage, the left adrenal is removed through an incision in the left flank.

Each method has advantages and disadvantages. The one stage technique, with an anterior approach, involves only one anaesthetic and probably only one incision. On the other hand, removal of the right adrenal may be technically difficult if the liver is enlarged. Also, the removal of both adrenals and ovaries in one operation is a big procedure for an ill patient to withstand. Many of these patients have pulmonary or pleural deposits and, as ATKINS et al. (1960) have shown, they are intolerant to the further burdens to their respiratory potential imposed by an upper abdominal incision.

The two stage technique, where the approach is through the bed of the eleventh or twelfth rib, is technically easier; also the removal of one gland at a time imposes less strain on the patient. But two anaesthetics are needed (usually the operations are done with about ten days' interval) and this again may involve an extra hazard to patients with metastatic pulmonary involvement.

No investigation has been carried out to decide which of the two techniques is preferable, nor probably will one ever be done. To all accounts, there is so little difference that, even if a randomised trial were carried out, the results would have little meaning.

One variation in technique has been championed by French surgeons and particularly by a group led by MARCEL DARGENT in Lyon. The operation entails first removing the right adrenal and both ovaries and then implanting a portion of the left adrenal gland into the spleen. By this means, the left adrenal remnant should obtain a new circulation from the splenic vessels, and any endocrine secretion from the implanted gland will be carried, via the portal circulation, to the liver. It is known that androgenic and oestrogenic hormones are broken down by the liver whilst corticosteroids can pass through the liver without being denatured. Therefore, following the implant, the patient should not need replacement therapy as she will still be secreting sufficient corticoids from the left adrenal remnant. Sex hormone secretion, although continuing, will have no physiological effect because the hormones will be immediately deactivated in the liver.

DARGENT et al. (1967) reported on 265 patients with advanced breast cancer who where considered for adrenal transplants. Only 143 of the patients (54 per cent) were found suitable for the operation—many were discarded because of large adrenal metastases or major involvement of the liver. The 143 patients who were accepted had a right adrenalectomy performed and a part of the left adrenal implanted into the spleen. Subsequently, seventeen of these patients developed immediate adrenal insufficiency; twenty of the patients developed a secondary adrenal insufficiency some weeks after the operation; a further forty six patients developed progressive late adrenal insufficiency as the cancer progressed. Only forty six patients lived from operation to death without replacement therapy. MAYER et al. (1967) reported that the remission rate in these 143 adrenal transplants was similar to that found in a parallel series of patients who had received bilateral adrenalectomy.

This technique has not been widely adopted and indeed is seldom practised outside France. Although ingenious in its conception, in practice it does not contribute materially to the management of patients with advanced breast cancer. Replacement therapy after bilateral adrenalectomy does not normally pose any major problems and, when only 54 per cent of those considered for transplant could be operated on and only 31 per cent of those operated on survived without going into adrenal failure, the effort involved does not seem justifiable.

INOKUCHI and IKEJIRI (1966) have described an operation with a similar principle in which the adrenal vein is anastomosed to a branch of the inferior mesenteric vein, the adrenal vein blood is thence carried directly to the liver through the portal system. They reported a significant remission rate (35 per cent) without going into details of the criteria of remission. Although none of their thirty two patients needed subsequently replacement therapy, the operation seems an unnecessary complication for a small return.

b) Hypophysectomy

a) By Surgery. There has been far more interest in designing alternative methods for pituitary ablation than for the removal of the adrenals. The various surgical techniques have been described in detail by SCHURR (1966) and THOMAS (1966). LUFT and OLIVECRONA (1953) used the transfrontal approach when they first tried hypophysectomy as a method of treatment for advanced breast cancer. This has remained the approach of choice when the operation has been in the hands of a neurosurgeon. The surgeon sees the pituitary fossa from an angle almost parallel to the floor of the anterior cranial fossa, and although there may be wide variations in the local anatomy which can hinder attempts at removal (see SCHURR, 1966), a complete hypophysectomy can be performed in almost all cases with remarkably little morbidity or mortality. The problem with the transfrontal approach is that it requires a particularly specialised expertise which can only be found in a neurosurgical unit. Even then, the best results will be obtained only if the unit is routinely and frequently carrying out hypophysectomies. There are hazards in the operation and aftercare which will be appreciated only by surgeons whose techniques has been shaped by the familiarity which is engendered by frequent repetition.

Not all breast clinics have recourse to such a neurosurgical service and attempts have been made to remove the pituitary by other methods. The most popular alternative operation has been the transphenoidal hypophysectomy, a procedure which is usually carried out by an Ear, Nose and Throat surgeon. Essentially this entails approaching the pituitary gland through the sphenoidal air sinus. This may be achieved by either a trans septal approach or a trans ethmoidal approach or by a modification of these. The principal complications of this method of pituitary ablation are bleeding, rhinorrhea and meningitis. On occasions, the haemorrhage may be so great that the operation has to be abandoned and a further attempt made a week to ten days later. More serious is the danger that, on occasions, all the gland may not be removed; the surgeon is working at a considerable depth and often under great difficulties and it may well be that portions of the pituitary gland remain after operation. The pituitary stalk is not divided in this operation and regrowth of the stalk may promote connections between pituitary remnants and the pituitary portal system. No evidence is available on the relative frequency of remissions following transfrontal and transphenoidal hypophysectomies but a controlled trial, comparing the two operations, is now being undertaken (HAYWARD and BULBROOK, 1968).

Pituitary stalk section probably has the same physiological effect as hypophysectomy. There is a massive infarct of the gland (SCHURR, 1966) and, providing a barrier (usually of acrylic resin) is placed over the pituitary fossa, the stalk does not regenerate. Pituitary stalk section interrupts the pituitary blood supply, apart from a small contribution obtained from the surrounding dura mater. Cortisone replacement therapy is required and the remission rates in patients with breast cancer may be similar to that obtained from hypophysectomy, although no comparative trials have been carried out. The operation is usually restricted to those patients in whom, because of local anatomical abnormalities, hypophysectomy by the transfrontal approach is found to be impossible.

β) By Irradiation. There has been widespread interest in developing a method of destroying the pituitary gland by ionising radiation. Vast doses of external radiation (70—100,000 rads) are needed for pituitary destruction and, when delivered by conventional apparatus, the degree of scatter inevitably means affecting surrounding structures such as the optic and oculomotor nerves. Apparatus which gives a very narrow beam of radiation has been tried in an attempt to confine the dose to the gland itself. LAWRENCE, TOBIAS and their group, working at the Laboratory of Medical Physics in Berkeley, California, have used an alpha particle beam or a proton beam from a cyclotron as a means of pituitary ablation. LAWRENCE (1967) reported the results on 176 patients with advanced breast cancer, treated by a heavy particle beam, and he claimed that about thirty four per cent had either a remission or the disease arrested. He stated that ablation could be achieved with a dose to the pituitary as low as 17,000 rads, delivered over a period of five days. But many of the patients in his series were receiving other forms of therapy at the same time and it is not possible to know how much of the effect was due to irradiation. Also, the full effect of the therapy takes a long time (about six months) to develop and this, coupled with the unavailability of the apparatus, makes heavy particle bombardment unlikely ever to be a serious contender as a method of pituitary ablation.

The possibilities of "internal irradiation", by implanting radioactive isotopes into the pituitary fossa, were first explored by FORREST and PEEBLES-BROWN (1955). After investigating the use of radon and 198 Au, both of which were eventually discarded because of side effects, they eventually elaborated a technique for the implantation of 90 Yttrium into the pituitary. Variations of this technique are now widely used and enable a pituitary ablation to be carried out with the minimum upset to the patient and with few side effects. The whole field of pituitary implantation has been reviewed in detail by FORREST (1959).

Most of the techniques are very similar and entail placing 90 Yttrium into the pituitary fossa, either within pellets, seeds or a screw. The latter method, in which the Yttrium is contained in the end of a screw which is inserted into the floor of the sella, has the advantage that the screw prevents subsequent cerebrospinal rhi-norrhoea. There are few complications from this technique and in 297 patients, FORREST and STEWART (1967) had only a 4 per cent mortality rate. Two per cent of their patients had rhinorrhoea and 4 per cent developed meningitis.

The question has always been whether pituitary ablation by Yttrium implantation gives an equivalent remission rate to that obtained by surgical hypophysectomy. In FORREST and STEWART's (1967) opinion, the response following surgical hypophys-ectomy is probably better than following Yttrium ablation. Moreover, they carried out three trials to assess the comparative value of Yttrium implantation and bilateral adrenalectomy with oophorectomy.

In one trial, including 78 patients, the results from screw implantation were compared with those from adrenalectomy; the patients were selected for the appro-priate treatment group by random sample. The remission rates from the two pro-cedures were very similar (21 per cent for implant, 25 per cent for adrenalectomy) but the duration of remission was longer following adrenalectomy (eighty-seven weeks compared with fifty weeks).

In the second trial, forty patients, who were deteriorating following a previous adrenalectomy, were further treated by a pituitary implant. Only two (5 per cent) had a further remission from the implant and both of these patients had previously responded to adrenalectomy.

In the third trial, twenty one patients, who were deteriorating following pituitary implants, were subsequently treated by bilateral adrenalectomy, and oophorectomy. Three (14 per cent) of these responded to adrenalectomy, two of which had pre-viously had a remission from implantation and one of which had failed to respond to implant.

FORREST's conclusions are worth quoting verbatim (FORREST and STEWART, 1967):

"It is clear from these results that Yttrium 90 implantation of the pituitary in its present form is not as consistently effective a method of suppressing endocrine function as is the surgical removal of the adrenals and ovaries. The extent of pitui-tary destruction assessed histologically post mortem in forty two patients support this conclusion; in only thirty (71 per cent) was complete or near complete (> 95 per cent) destruction observed."

5. Endocrine Changes after Ablation

Studies on the changes that result from adrenalectomy or hypophysectomy have had two principal aims. Firstly, to see whether any specific post operative hormone pattern is associated with a favourable response and, secondly, to find an accurate guide (particularly in the case of hypophysectomy) to the completeness of the operation. A detailed account of the endocrine changes that follow ablation has been given by BULBROOK and STRONG (1959). The effects of the operations on other factors such as electrolyte balance and water metabolism, etc., have been well catalogued (see SCHURR, 1966; PEARSON and RAY, 1958) and will not be mentioned further.

a) Postoperative Hormone Levels and Response

If the aim of ablation is to remove all sources of sex hormones, a logical explanation of failure to respond might be found in the continued presence after operation of small quantities of these hormones in the urine. This has not proved to be so. Although investigations of postoperative urine specimens have revealed measurable amounts of hormones on many occasions, their presence has not correlated with a failure to respond. BULBROOK et al. (1958 a and b) described the presence of measurable amounts of oestrogen in the urine of patients who had had a bilateral adrenalectomy with oophorectomy for advanced breast cancer. No correlation could be demonstrated between the continued oestrogen excretion and the response to operation. Similar findings have been noted with posthypophysectomy gonadotrophin and 17-oxosteroid levels (BECK et al., 1966).

It is known that the adrenal cortex atrophies after hypophysectomy and JANTET et al. (1963) have studied the extent of this atrophy in post hypophysectomy patients and controls. Adrenocortical atrophy was marked in the hypophysectomy patients but again it did not correlate with response to treatment. Sometimes only minor degrees of atrophy were found in patients who had had a successful response.

BULBROOK (1965) described how these unexpected findings caused considerable controversy amongst workers in this field and how a lot of unnecessary work was carried out to substantiate claims that when seen retrospectively were quite unimportant. The truth of the matter seems to be that, within limits, there is no association between response to adrenalectomy or hypophysectomy and the continued excretion of small amounts of hormones in the urine. Measurable amounts of hormone can be present in successful cases, whilst zero figures will be recorded in patients who have failed to respond. There is probably a level of circulating hormones to which the tumour cells are sensitive and any amount below this will have little or no physiological effect. The majority of ablative procedures, although possibly incomplete, will result in levels below this physiological limit; low titres of hormone will continue to be excreted but this excretion will have little practical importance.

b) The Measurement of Completeness of Operation

Although the presence postoperatively of trace amounts of hormones in the urine does not necessarily mean that ablation has been a failure, it can still be important to know that the operation has been complete. There have been occasions in which adrenalectomy has been successful after a failed hypophysectomy and vice versa (see for instance FORREST and STEWART, 1967). But this happens infrequently and a second operation would never be advisable unless the surgeon had firm evidence of the incompleteness of the first procedure.

There is unlikely to be doubt of the completeness of bilateral adrenalectomy. Adrenal activity may continue but this is probably due to ectopic adrenal rests which are known to be present in certain cases and may be undetected at the time of operation. There is some doubt of the functional ability of these rests but on occasions they can probably secrete significant amounts of hormones. Following withdrawal of cortisone, an ACTH stimulation test should reveal the presence of active adrenal tissue by the detection of raised plasma cortisol levels.

The measurement of the completeness of hypophysectomy is more frequently required but less easy to carry out. There are many possible tests of continuing pituitary activity and these have been described in detail by LORAINE (1966). The development of an Addisonian crisis following the withdrawal of cortisone gives an indication that probably 90 per cent of the gland has been removed but it is a manoeuvre which is seldom justified. The measurement of thyroid activity by the uptake of ^{131}I is a sensitive indication of pituitary activity; a reduced uptake is noted almost immediately after hypophysectomy. Similarly, gonadotrophin levels fall soon after the pituitary gland has been removed, although physiological amounts may occasionally be measured in the urine up to two to three weeks later. BECK et al. (1966) consider that a combination of low gonadotrophin output and a low ^{131}I uptake gives the best indication of completeness of operation, although the presence of small remnants of remaining pituitary tissue would not be excluded.

The development of a radioimmunological assay for the measurement of growth hormone levels in human plasma (HUNTER and GREENWOOD, 1964) has enabled a more accurate assessment to be made of the completeness of hypophysectomy. Plasma levels of growth hormone fall to zero after total pituitary ablation. Following a 24-hour withdrawal of cortisone, the administration of small doses of insulin will result in the appearance of detectable amounts of growth hormone in the plasma if the pituitary removal has not been total (GREENWOOD, 1967). This test promises to be of value in comparing the different techniques of pituitary ablation.

Summary and Conclusions

1. In about 30 per cent of patients with advanced breast cancer, adrenalectomy or hypophysectomy will cause all lesions to improve for at least six months.

2. Under ideal conditions, hypophysectomy gives better results and a longer period of survival than adrenalectomy. Hypophysectomy is to be preferred when skilled facilities are available for carrying out the operation completely and with little morbidity and mortality. When such facilities are not available, adrenalectomy is the operation of choice.

3. The response rate from ablation is approximately twice that from hormone therapy. The response from ablation is not due to the steroids administered as replacement therapy. A "medical adrenalectomy", resulting from administering corticosteroids to patients with intact adrenals, does not give as good a response as surgical adrenalectomy.

4. The response rate following ablation is lower if previous hormone therapy has been given. Only 60 per cent of patients subjected to hormone therapy as a first treatment for recurrence, will survive to ablation.

5. Early ablation, performed without an initial trial of hormone therapy, does not give an improvement in remission or survival. Adrenalectomy and hypophysectomy should be reserved for patients with established advanced or metastatic disease on whom simpler methods of treatment have failed.

6. A transfrontal hypophysectomy is the surest way of effecting a total pituitary ablation. The transphenoidal operation may achieve as much in skilled hands. 90 Yttrium implants probably leave a significant amount of viable pituitary tissue behind in some cases.

7. Tests of completeness of operation are rarely of practical use in ablative surgery. It is seldom, if ever justified to recommend hypophysectomy if adrenalectomy has failed or vice versa.

References

ATKINS, H. J. B.: In: Clinical evaluation in breast cancer. Ed. J. L. HAYWARD and R. D. BULBROOK. London-New York: Academic Press 1966 a, p. 214.
— Carcinoma of the breast. Ann. R. Coll. Surg. 38, 133 (1966 b).
— FALCONER, M. A., HAYWARD, J. L., MACLEAN, K. S.: Adrenalectomy and hypophysectomy for advanced cancer of the breast. A comparative study. Lancet 1957 I, 489.
— — — — SCHURR, P. H.: The timing of adrenalectomy and of hypophysectomy in the treatment of advanced breast cancer. Lancet 1966 I, 827.
— — — — — ARMITAGE, P.: Adrenalectomy and hypophysectomy for advanced cancer of the breast. Lancet 1960 I, 1148.
BECK, J. C., BLAIR, A. J., GRIFFITHS, M. M., ROSENFELD, M. W., MCGARRY, E. E.: In search of hormonal factors as an aid in predicting the outcome of breast carcinoma. In: Proc. Sixth Canadian Cancer Conference. Pergamon Press 1966, p. 3.
BULBROOK, R. D.: Hormone assays in human breast cancer. Vitam. and Horm. 23, 329 (1965).
— GREENWOOD, F. C., HADFIELD, G. J., SCOWEN, E. F.: Adrenalectomy in breast cancer. An attempt to correlate clinical results with oestrogen production. Brit. med. J. I, 12 (1958 a).
— — — — Hypophysectomy in breast cancer. An attempt to correlate clinical results with oestrogen production. Brit. med. J. I, 15 (1958 b).
— STRONG, J. A.: Hormone studies in breast cancer. In: Cancer 6. Ed.: R. W. RAVEN. London: Butterworth 1959, p. 215.
BYRON, JR., R. J.: Randomised adrenalectomies in advanced breast cancer. In: Major Endocrine Surgery for the treatment of cancer of the breast in advanced stages. Eds.: M. DARGENT and CL. ROMIEU. Lyon: Simep Editions 1967, p. 253.
CHABANIER, H., PUECH, P., LOBO-ONELL, C., LELU, E.: Hypophyse et diabète (à propos de l'ablation d'une hypophyse normale dans un cas de diabète grave). Presse méd. 44, 986 (1936).
CUTLER, M.: Tumours of the breast. Philadelphia-Montreal: Lippincott 1962.
CUTLER, S. J.: In: Clinical evaluation in breast cancer. Eds.: J. L. HAYWARD and R. D. BULBROOK. London-New York: Academic Press 1966, p. 214.
DAO, T. L.: Adrenalectomy for mammary cancer; a review. Quart. Rev. Surg. Obst. Gynec. 17, 75 (1960).
— NEMOTO, T.: An evaluation of adrenalectomy and androgen in disseminated mammary carcinoma. Surg. Gynec. Obstet. 121, 1257 (1965).
— — BROSS, I. D. J.: A controlled, randomised, comparative study of early and late adrenalectomy in women with advanced breast cancer. In: Prognostic Factors in Breast Cancer. Eds.: A. P. M. FORREST and P. B. KUNKLER. Edinburgh: Livingstone 1968, p. 177.
— TAN, E., BROOKS, V.: A comparative evaluation of adrenalectomy and cortisone in the treatment of advanced mammary carcinoma. Cancer 14, 1259 (1961).
DARGENT, M., MAYER, M., LOMBARD, R.: Modalités techniques de la chirurgie surrénalienne: surrénalectomie bilatérale d'emblée ou en deux temps transplantation surréno-splénique. In: Major Endocrine Surgery for the treatment of Cancer of the Breast in advanced stages. Eds.: M. DARGENT and CL. ROMIEU. Lyon: Simep Éditions 1967, p. 61.
DRAGSTEDT, L. R.: Immediate oophorectomy and adrenalectomy in metastatic breast cancer. Proc. Nat. Acad. Sci. 47, 1069 (1961).
— HUMPHREYS, E. M., DRAGSTEDT II, L. R.: Prophylactic bilateral adrenalectomy and oophorectomy for advanced cancer of the breast. Surgery 47, 885 (1960).
FORREST, A. P. M.: Radiation hypophysectomy. In: Cancer 6. Ed.: R. W. RAVEN. London: Butterworth 1959, p. 274.

FORREST, A. P. M., PEEBLES BROWN, D. A.: Pituitary-radon implant for breast cancer. Lancet I, 1054 (1955).
— STEWART, H. J.: Technical problems and results of Yttrium hypophysectomy. In: Major endocrine surgery for the treatment of cancer of the breast in advanced stages. Eds.: M. DARGENT and CL. ROMIEU: Lyon: Simep Éditions 1967, p. 89.
— — BENSON, E. A., KER, H., JONES, V., KUNKLER, P. B., CAMPBELL, H.: Controlled studies in advanced breast cancer. In: Prognostic Factors in Breast Cancer. Eds.: A. P. M. FORREST and P. B. KUNKLER. Edinburgh: Livingstone 1968, p. 186.
FRACCHIA, A. A., RANDALL, H. T., FARROW, J. H.: The results of adrenalectomy in advanced breast cancer in 500 consecutive patients. Surg. Gynec. Obstet. 125, 747 (1967).
GORDAN, G. S.: Why are the reported results of hypophysectomy so variable? In: Current concepts in breast cancer. Eds.: A. SEGALOFF, K. K. MEYER, and S. DE BAKEY. Baltimore: Williams and Wilkins 1967, p. 342.
GREENWOOD, F. C.: Biological problems regarding hormonal surgery. In: Major endocrine surgery in the treatment of cancer of the breast in advanced stages. Eds.: M. DARGENT and CL. ROMIEU. Lyon: Simep Éditions 1967, p. 199.
HAYWARD, J. L.: Assessment of response to treatment at Guy's Hospital Breast Clinic. In: Clinical Evaluation in Breast Cancer. Eds.: J. L. HAYWARD and R. D. BULBROOK. London-New York: Academic Press 1966, pp. 131, 285.
— The place of adrenalectomy and hyophysectomy in the treatment of advanced breast cancer. In: Major Endocrine Surgery for the treatment of cancer of the breast in advanced stages. Eds.: M. DARGENT and CL. ROMIEU. Lyon: Simep Éditions 1967, p. 243.
— BULBROOK, R. D.: Urinary steroids and prognosis in breast cancer. In: Prognostic Factors in Breast Cancer. Eds.: A. P. M. FORREST and P. B. KUNKLER. Edinburgh: Livingstone 1968, p. 383.
HUGGINS, C., DAO, T. L.-Y.: Adrenalectomy and Oophorectomy in treatment of advanced carcinoma of the breast. J. Amer. med. Ass. 151, 1388 (1953).
HUNTER, W. M., GREENWOOD, F. C.: A radio-immunoelectrophoretic assay for human growth hormone. Biochem. J. 91, 43 (1964).
INOKUCHI, K., IKEJIRI, T.: Suprarenal-inferior mesenteric venous shunt for advanced carcinoma of the breast. Arch. Surg. 92, 853 (1966).
JANTET, B., CROCKER, D. W., SHIRAKI, M., MOORE, F. D.: Adrenal suppression in disseminated carcinoma of the breast. New Engl. J. Med. 269, 1 (1963).
Joint Committee on Endocrine Ablative Procedures in Disseminated Mammary Carcinoma. Adrenalectomy and Hypophysectomy in disseminated mammary carcinoma. J. Amer. med. Ass. 175, 787 (1961).
KENNEDY, B. J., FRENCH, L.: Hypophysectomy in advanced breast cancer. Amer. J. Surg. 110, 411 (1965).
LAWRENCE, J. H.: Heavy particle irradiation to the pituitary in metastatic breast cancer. In: Major Endocrine Surgery for the treatment of cancer of the breast in advanced stages. Eds.: M. DARGENT and CL. ROMIEU. Lyon: Simep Éditions 1967, p. 89.
LORAINE, J. A.: Clinical tests of anterior pituitary activity. In: The pituitary gland 2. Eds.: G. W. HARRIS and B. T. DONOVAN. London: Butterworth 1966, p. 545.
LUFT, R., OLIVECRONA, H.: Experiences with hypophysectomy in man. J. Neurosurg. 10, 301 (1953).
— — IKKOS, D., NILSSON, L. B., MOSSBERG, H.: Hypophysectomy in the management of metastatic carcinoma of the breast. In: Endocrine aspects of breast cancer. Eds.: A. R. CURRIE and C. W. F. ILLINGWORTH. Edinburgh-London: Livingstone 1959, p. 27.
MACDONALD, I.: Endocrine ablation in disseminated mammary carcinoma. Surg. Gynec. Obstet. 115, 215 (1962).
MAYER, M., DARGENT, M., POMMATAU, E., SAEZ, S.: Résultats de la transplantation surréno-splénique associée à la surrénalectomie droite et à l'ovariectomie dans le traitement du cancer du sein en phase avancée chez la femme. In: Major Endocrine Surgery for the treatment of cancer of the breast in advanced stages. Eds.: M. DARGENT and CL. ROMIEU. Lyon: Simep Éditions 1967, p. 67.
PATEY, D. H.: Early (prophylactic) oophorectomy and adrenalectomy in carcinoma of the breast, an interim report. Brit. J. Cancer XIV, 457 (1960).

PEARSON, O. H., RAY, B. S.: Physiological effects of adrenalectomy and hypophysectomy. In: Endocrine aspects of breast cancer. Eds.: A. R. CURRIE and C. F. W. ILLINGWORTH. Edinburgh-London: Livingstone 1958, p. 90.

— — A comparison of the results of adrenalectomy and hypophysectomy in carcinoma of the breast. In: Cancer 6. Ed.: R. W. RAVEN. London: Butterworth 1959, p. 335.

— — Hypophysectomy in the treatment of metastatic mammary cancer. Amer. J. Surg. 99, 544 (1960).

PROHASKA, J.: Mammary carcinoma metastases. Response to Endocrine Ablative Surgery. In: Major Endocrine Surgery for the treatment of cancer of the breast in advanced stages. Eds.: M. DARGENT and CL. ROMIEU. Lyon: Simep Éditions 1967, p. 37.

RAY, B. S., PEARSON, O. H.: Surgical hypophysectomy in the treatment of advanced cancer of the breast. In: Endocrine Aspects of breast cancer. Eds.: A. R. CURRIE and C. F. W. ILLINGWORTH. Edinburgh-London: Livingstone 1958, p. 36.

SCHURR, P. H.: Techniques and effects of hypophysectomy, pituitary stalk section and pituitary transplantation in man. In: The Pituitary gland, Vol. 2. Eds.: G. E. HARRIS and B. T. DONOVAN. London: Butterworth 1966, p. 22.

SEGALOFF, A.: Assessment of response to treatment by the Co-operative Breast Cancer Group. In: Clinical Evaluation in Breast Cancer. Eds.: J. L. HAYWARD and R. D. BULBROOK. London-New York: Academic Press 1966, pp. 125, 275.

SELLWOOD, R. A., DAVEY, J., DEELEY, T. J., GALASKO, C. S. B., FOTHERBY, K., LI, J., BURN, J. I.: A clinical trial to compare early and late pituitary ablation in advanced cancer of the breast. Brit. J. Surg. 55, 870 (1968).

STRONG J. A.: Hormonal control of cancer. Proc. roy. Soc. Med. 56, 665 (1963).

THOMAS, K. E.: Trans-sphenoidal hypophysectomy. J. Laryng. 80, 804 (1966).

Chapter 4

Tests of Prediction

Since adrenalectomy and hypophysectomy were first used successfully in the treatment of advanced breast cancer, there has been a need for an accurate method of predicting those patients most likely to succeed. The success rate from these operations, when judged on strict objective criteria, is little more than 30 per cent. These are major operations which are only palliative in their effect and usually carried out on patients who are in the terminal stages of a lethal disease. Accurate prediction is essential, and yet has still not been attained. In spite of the very considerable amount of work carried out by a large number of investigators, no precise and practical method of prediction has yet been suggested.

The whole field of prediction has been reviewed in great detail by FAIRGRIEVE (1965). Further aspects have been discussed by McCALISTER et al. (1961), BULBROOK (1965) and BECK et al. (1966).

1. Clinical Methods

The search for factors which may predict the response of patients with advanced breast cancer to subsequent adrenalectomy or hypophysectomy, has been most active in the clinical field. A large amount of data is now available on patients who have undergone these operations, and these data can be compared retrospectively with the patients' subsequent fate.

a) The Histology of the Tumour

A reasonable assumption would be that the histology of the tumour would correlate with response to endocrine ablation. If the hormone responsiveness of a tumour is a feature derived from its parent tissue, then the more akin the tumour is to its tissue of origin, the more likely it is to be hormone responsive. This means that the tumour which is highly differentiated, mimicking as closely as possible the ductal and acinar pattern of the normal breast, would be the most likely to be hormone responsive and hence most likely to respond in its advanced stages to alterations in the hormonal environment by adrenalectomy or hypophysectomy. Indeed, in one of the first papers published on the results of adrenalectomy (HUGGINS and DAO, 1954), an association was described between tumour differentiation and response, but these preliminary observations have not been confirmed in subsequent publications by other workers (for instance ALLEN et al., 1957; LIPSETT et al., 1957; BLOCK et al., 1959). Even the most anaplastic of tumours can respond well to hormone manipulation whilst those that are highly differentiated can prove resistant.

Using mitotic and resting cell counts as an indication of tumour activity, WOLFF (1957) compared cell differentiation in biopsy specimens with the patient's subsequent response to ablation. No correlation was detected.

With current histological techniques, the microscopical features of a tumour seem to be of no help in the prediction of response.

b) Macroscopical Features of the Tumour

There have been some indications that response varies according to the dominant site of metastases. For instance, it is frequently reported that patients with visceral metastases fare badly after ablation compared with those with locally advanced tumours or those having bony metastases (see for example McCALISTER et al., 1961). On the other hand, other investigators (for example PEARSON and RAY, 1960) have not been able to demonstrate any correlation between the site of metastases and response. The truth probably lies somewhere between the two. As a result of the destruction of essential tissue, patients with severe liver, lung or brain involvement are probably more at risk at operation. If they survive, and even if there is some degree of remission, the amount of normal tissue remaining in these organs may not be sufficient to maintain life for long.

If all other factors are equals the presence of metastases at any particular site should not preclude an operation. After adrenalectomy or hypophysectomy multiple metastases in the liver or lungs can disappear to give many years of normal life.

c) Response to Previous Hormone Therapy

There is conflicting evidence on the predictive value of response to previous hormone therapy. PEARSON and RAY (1960) demonstrated some correlation between the response to androgen therapy and subsequent hypophysectomy. Conversely, DAO and NEMOTO (1965) concluded that the response to hormonal therapy was not a

Table 12. *The response to hormone therapy expressed according to the subsequent response to ablation.* (ATKINS et al., 1966)

Response to hormones	Subsequent response to operation		
	Success	Intermediate	Failure
Success (9 cases)	1	5	3
Intermediate (18 cases)	6	5	7
Failure (30 cases)	6	6	18

reliable guide to the subsequent response to adrenalectomy. ATKINS et al. (1966), in their trial comparing early with late ablation in the treatment of advanced breast cancer, reported on fifty seven patients who were treated by both hormone therapy and ablation. Table 12 shows the response of these patients, both to hormones and to adrenalectomy or hypophysectomy. There is no correlation, and indeed only one patient had a successful response to both forms of treatment. On the other hand, the

actual administration of hormones, irrespective of response, seems to affect the remission rate following subsequent endocrine ablation. Both DAO and NEMOTO (1965)
and ATKINS et al. (1966) observed that patients who have received hormone therapy
have a noticeably lower response to subsequent ablation than do patients who have
had no hormone therapy before operation.

d) The Response to Previous Castration (see also pages 14—15)

It would be unlikely that the response to castration more accurate prediction than
the response to hormone therapy, yet this may be the case. Many workers (see for
instance PEARSON and RAY, 1960, for hypophysectomy and BLOCK et al., 1959, would
give for adrenalectomy) have noted a positive correlation between a successful response
to ovarian ablation and a successful response to adrenalectomy or hypophysectomy.
Indeed, there are many physicians who refuse to recommend a patient for adrenalectomy or hypophysectomy unless a good response to oophorectomy or ovarian irradiation has previously been noted. Nevertheless, this aid to prediction must be of
limited value only. Firstly, it cannot help if the metastases occur when the patient
is postmenopausal. Secondly, no information will be available in those younger patients who have had their ovaries removed as a prophylactic measure at mastectomy.
FAIRGRIEVE (1965) states as his personal observation that the response to ovarian
ablation, as a criterion for subsequent response to adrenalectomy or hypophysectomy,
is applicable in less than ten per cent of patients. The remaining 90 per cent either
have undergone oophorectomy prior to the onset of the disease, or have had an
oophorectomy a year or two after the menopause, or have had a prophylactic
oophorectomy at mastectomy, or have undergone oophorectomy when the metastases
were hidden or symptomless and a valid judgement of the result is not possible.

Although FAIRGRIEVE felt that the response to oophorectomy was rarely applicable for prediction, there are obviously many who find it a useful measure. More
work is needed on this subject. Not only is it important to know more about the
value of ovarian ablation as a tool for prediction but also this information may
affect the place and timing of ovarian surgery in the management of breast disease.

e) The Free Period

In this context, the free period is defined as the time interval between mastectomy
and recurrence. The length of this interval gives some information on the growth
rate of the tumour. If the free period is short, the tumour is rapidly growing and
the prognosis is poor. Conversely, if the free period is long, the tumour may be slow
growing and the patient have a better prognosis. In addition, patients with a long
free period seem to respond better to adrenalectomy or hypophysectomy than patients with a short free period. (See for example MACDONALD, 1962; PEARSON and
RAY, 1960.) It is not known why slowly growing tumours tend to be hormone
responsive whilst rapidly growing tumours do not respond. It seems to have no connection with the degree of anaplasia of the tumour (see page 52), although anaplastic
tumours usually grow rapidly.

Unlike the factors so far discussed, the free period seems to be of practical use
in prediction. HAYWARD and BULBROOK (1968) chose an arbitrary time of two years.
Those patients having a free period of longer than two years stand a good chance

of responding to ablation, whilst those having a free period of less than two years are likely to fare badly.

The disadvantage of this method of prediction is that many patients will not have had a mastectomy—nor indeed any potentially curative treatment for the primary disease—and hence an estimation of the length of the free period is not possible. An alternative is to assess the total duration of the disease up to ablation. BLOCK et al. (1959) showed that in patients who responded to adrenalectomy, the average duration from first symptom to adrenalectomy was 63.3 months, whereas in those who failed to respond, the duration was 31.2 months. HUGGINS and DAO (1954) and LIPSETT et al. (1957) reported similar findings. The disadvantage of an estimate of the total duration of the disease is that reliance has to be placed on the patient's statement of when she first noticed her symptoms; this may be subject to considerable error. Also, total duration must be affected by the period during which other therapies have been tried. Patients who have been treated previously by oestrogens, androgens or steroids will probably have a longer total duration of their disease than those who are recommended immediate ablation. It has been shown that previous treatment by hormones decreased the response rate to adrenalectomy or hypophysectomy (ATKINS et al., 1966; DAO and NEMOTO, 1965) and hence the use of hormone treatment may affect the predictive value of the length of time from first symptom to ablation. The effect of hormone therapy may explain the finding of McCALISTER et al. (1961) who showed that patients who had ablative surgery within six months of the disease becoming "uncontrolled" had a higher response rate (51 per cent) than patients who had their operation more than six months from the disease becoming "uncontrolled" (30 per cent). The delay in the latter group may well have been due to the patients being treated with hormones. McCALISTER and his colleagues were unable to show any correlation between response and total duration of disease.

f) Menopausal Status

There seems to be some controversy on the exact effect of the menopausal status on a patient's response to ablation. The position is particularly confused because most reported series include patients who have had their periods stopped by oophorectomy or ovarian irradiation or whose periods have stopped as a result of androgen therapy. Difficulties also arise in categorising patients who have had a previous hysterectomy with retention of the ovaries. When those patients whose menopausal status is accurately known are allotted to pre- and post-menopausal groups, little difference can be detected in the response rate to ablation. It is only when patients who are just menopausal are considered as a separate entitiy that a difference emerges. BULBROOK and HAYWARD (1967) have shown that the response rate to adrenalectomy or hypophysectomy is very low when the operations are performed on patients who are within six years of the menopause. Only five out of forty four (11 per cent) postmenopausal patients responded, compared with twenty seven out of seventy three (37 per cent) premenopausal patients and fourteen out of fifty three (26 per cent) patients who were more than five years postmenopausal. The menopausal status can be put to greater practical use as a predictive measure when hormone assays are taken into account (see below).

2. Hormone Assays

For some time, the principal responsibility for finding an accurate method for predicting the results of adrenalectomy or hypophysectomy has lain in the hands of the biochemists. It has been assumed that the hormone responsiveness of a tumour is either a specific property of that tumour, derived from its parent tissue, or acquired and determined by the environment in which the tumour is growing; a third and more likely possibility, is that it is a combination of both factors. On the hypothesis that at least some of the tumour's responsiveness derives from its environment, for many years and with varying degrees of success, investigators have attempted to assay hormone levels in the blood and urine of patients with breast cancer. These assays have been beset with methodological difficulties, and the introduction of new and more specific methods of measurement has meant that much of the earlier work has had to be discarded. To date, most hormone assays have been carried out on urine samples; these assays gave information on the excretory pattern of hormones, but not necessarily on the levels in the blood stream and hence the amounts available to the breast and breast tumour. Methods for the accurate assay of hormone levels in the blood are now becoming available and probably herald a whole new era in hormone research. In the meanwhile, the results from urinary steroid estimations are giving valuable, if inadequate, information on the hormonal environment of patients with breast cancer. In an attempt to find some pattern which would correlate with response to adrenalectomy or hypophysectomy, the assays have usually been carried out on pre-operative urine specimens. This work has had some success and has stimulated physicians and scientists to believe that when more sophisticated techniques of measurement are available, this field of research could be of fundamental importance in understanding the initiation and growth of breast cancer.

a) Oestrogen Assays

Until a few years ago, it seemed that investigations of the oestrogenic status of patients with breast cancer was likely to be most rewarding. It had always been assumed that breast tumours were "oestrogen dependent" and that if accurate methods for measuring natural oestrogens were available a correlation would be demonstrated between oestrogen levels and tumour behaviour. Almost simultaneously, BROWN (1955) and BAULD (1956) developed methods for the accurate chemical estimation of small amounts of oestrone, oestriol and oestradiol 17β in human urine. The stage seemed set for a major advance in the understanding of the mechanics of hormonal control in breast cancer. But this never came. Many investigators measured the urinary oestrogen levels in patients before or after adrenalectomy or hypophysectomy (for instance, BROWN et al., 1959; BULBROOK et al., 1958 a and b) but with little advantage. BULBROOK and his colleagues (1958 b) showed that patients responding to hypophysectomy tended to have a low preoperative oestrogen excretion and patients who did not respond tended to have high levels, but they were unable to demonstrate a similar correlation with adrenalectomy (BULBROOK et al., 1958 a). Similarly, continuing oestrogen excretion after operation did not exclude a remission. Admittedly, BLOCK et al. (1959) reported that response to adrenalectomy could be predicted by measuring the preoperative levels of urinary oestrogen; patients with high titres had a successful response to the operation and patients with low titres failed to respond. BLOCK and his colleagues believed that a remission would be obtained in two thirds to three quarters of the patients if the operation was restricted to those who excreted relatively large amounts of urinary oestrogens. But this was an isolated report in which only twenty seven patients were studied and the findings have not been confirmed. It is generally accepted that the measurement of oestrogens in urine, by the techniques now in use, will give no useful information on which the prediction of the response to subsequent ablation can be based. This does not necessarily mean that the end of the story has been reached. There are many difficulties still to be overcome. For instance, in a premenopausal woman, a meaningful assessment of her oestrogen excretion can only result from determinations carried out right through a menstrual cycle—in fact measurements should probably continue throughout two or three menstrual cycles. If many patients were involved, such a study would be very difficult with the present analytical methods. Similarly, in postmenopausal women, accurate measurements of the very low excretion of oestrogen is difficult and little credence can be given to many of the reported values. Perhaps the greatest errors have been due to the heterogeneity of the patients who have been investigated. As BULBROOK (1965) has pointed out, some of the authors studied extremely mixed populations and usually only small numbers of patients.

With improvement in methods, oestrogen estimations may yet have a part to play in the study of the hormonal basis of breast cancer. To date, they have contributed little and at present have no place in predicting the response to adrenalectomy or hypophysectomy.

b) Androgens and Corticosteroids

In 1957, ALLEN, HAYWARD and MERIVALE published a report on the measurement of urinary androgen and corticosteroid metabolites in fifteen patients with advanced mammary cancer who subsequently were subjected to adrenalectomy with oophorectomy or to hypophysectomy. A total seventy two hour urine collection had been collected from each patient before operation and, on aliquots from this specimen, the 11-deoxy-17-oxosteroids (products of androgen metabolism) and the 11-oxy-17-oxosteroids (products of cortisol metabolism) were estimated. A comparison was then made between the relative amounts of these substances in each patient and her subsequent response to adrenalectomy or hypophysectomy. A correlation was noted when the relative amounts of the 11-deoxy and 11-oxy-17-oxosteroids were expressed as a simple ratio. In those patients who benefited from the subsequent operation, the ratio was greater than one and the excretion pattern approximated to that found in healthy subjects. In those patients who did not benefit, the ratio was less than one.

This work was severely and justifiably criticised—principally for the methods used in the steroid analyses. In particular, the hot acid hydrolysis used in the extraction of the urine, probably converted many of the 11-hydroxy compounds into $\Delta 9$—11 dehydration artefacts which would have been indistinguishable from the 11-deoxy compounds. In addition, possibly up to 80 per cent of the dehydroepiandrosterone would have been destroyed. Nevertheless—and taking into account the deficiencies of the method—the findings suggested two principles which have since been confirmed by other workers using more sophisticated assay techniques. Firstly, certain urinary hormone patterns correlated with success or failure to endocrine ablation (that is high androgen, low corticoid with success, low androgen, high corticoid with failure). Secondly, successful response to adrenalectomy or hypophysectomy was associated with normal hormonal excretion, and failure to respond to these operations with an abnormal hormonal excretion.

These findings of ALLEN et al. (1957) were subsequently reported in Glasgow at a meeting on the endocrine aspects of breast cancer. At the same meeting, a paper was presented by PLANTIN and his colleagues (1958) in which they also compared the 11-deoxy or 11-oxy-17-oxosteroid excretion with the response to endocrine ablation. They used more reliable methods of assay than ALLEN et al. (1957) but were unable to report a similar correlation. Furthermore, HOBKIRK and FORREST (1957) were also unable to find a correlation between assays of the fractionated 17-oxosteroids and the response to endocrine ablation, but again both their clinical material and their biochemical methods were different.

Nevertheless, in 1959, at a meeting of the Endocrine Society in Edinburgh, a further paper presented by different authors again described a close association between the excretion of androgen and corticosteroid metabolites and response to adrenalectomy and hypophysectomy. In this paper, HAYWARD, BULBROOK and GREENWOOD (1961) reported on a series of forty one patients, on whom they had carried out a wide range of hormone estimations. Table 13 shows the substances that

Table 13. *Substances measured and methods used.* (BULBROOK et al., 1960)

Substance	Method
Oestrone Oestradiol-17β Oestriol	BROWN, BULBROOK and GREENWOOD, 1957
17-oxosteroids 17-OHCS	NORYMBERSKI et al., 1955
Dehydroepiandrosterone Androsterone Aetiocholanolone 11-oxy-17-oxosteroids	KELLIE and WADE, 1957
Pregnanediol	KLOPPER, MICHIE and BROWN, 1955
Gonadotrophin	LORAINE and BROWN, 1956

were assayed on a five day pool of urine collected before operation and also lists the methods that were used for each assay. The estimations were carried out "blind" in that the results of the hormone assays were not revealed until the operations of adrenalectomy or hypophysectomy had been carried out and the response of the patients was known. By assaying such a large number of hormones, an attempt was made to measure as many representatives as possible of the products of ovarian, adrenal and pituitary activity which might conceivably have some effect on the behaviour of breast cancer. The design of the experiment also gives some indication that at that time there was little insight into which hormones or groups of hormones might correlate with response. The authors decided that if they measured as many steroid hormones as the available methods made possible, there was a good chance of identifying those compounds which might be of practical use in the management of breast cancer—providing such compounds existed.

This blanket type of approach to a problem can be very dangerous. The aim here was to find a correlation between the assays of one or more substance and the response to treatment. If these assays varied directly with response, a statistical test would be applied to see if this variation was significant. A probability of 0.05 would be acceptable, indicating that the observed results would have occurred by chance on one occasion in twenty or, expressed another way, if twenty substances were measured there would be an even chance that one of them would vary significantly with response. By choosing to measure about ten compounds (although admittedly some were closely related), HAYWARD and his colleagues probably stood a 2:1 chance of finding in one of them a correlation with response, significant at the five per cent level. In the event, they found a correlation with response in two of the compounds or groups of compounds measured. Table 14 gives details of the mean hormone excretion levels for their patients. There was no significant correlation between the oestrogens, total 17-oxosteroids, 11-oxy-17-oxosteroids, pregnanediol and gonadotrophin fractions and subsequent response to operation. But the mean aetiocholanolone level was significantly higher and the mean 17-hydroxy cortico-

Table 14. *Mean steroid excretion levels in patients showing regression, no change and failure to adrenalectomy or hypophysectomy.* (HAYWARD et al., 1961)

		Regression	No change	Failure
Number of cases		12	11	18
Total 17-oxosteroids	} (mg)	4.4	3.9	3.8
17-OHCS		7.1	8.0	11.0
Total oestrogen	} (µg)	8.8	7.1	9.1
Oestrone		2.6	1.7	2.3
Oestriol		5.3	4.7	5.9
DHA		217	137	154
Androsterone		718	450	584
Aetiocholanolone		805	495	543
11-oxy-17-oxosteroids		861	787	745
Pregnanediol		570	600	550
Gonadotrophin (HMG units)		6.5	2.5	12.0

steroids (17-OHCS) were significantly lower in the regression group compared with the failure group. The differences were significant at $P = 0.05$.

The question was raised whether these differences could be used in a prospective study to predict a patient's likely response to endocrine ablation. Unfortunately, this was not so, mainly because the overlap of values in the regression and failure groups was such that hormone levels in an individual patient would have little meaning. But it was pointed out that it would theoretically have been possible to predict accurately the response of 80 per cent of the patients in the small series under study by using an arbitrary ratio of the 17-OHCS to aetiocholanolone.

These results, although measuring slightly different compounds and using different methods, tended to confirm ALLEN and her colleagues' (1957) previous suggestion that levels of urinary androgen and corticoid metabolites correlate with response to adrenalectomy or hypophysectomy. What was also becoming clear was that the measurement of these hormones alone was unlikely to give a completely accurate forecast of response. Other parameters would probably be required and it was suggested that consideration of age, menopausal status and previous hormone therapy might sharpen the accuracy of prediction. Initially, more patients were needed for study to ensure that the observed association between hormone levels and response was not due to chance. If confirmation was obtained, the application of the results to the clinical management of patients would have to be considered.

A further report was soon published (BULBROOK, GREENWOOD and HAYWARD, 1960). The urinary oestrogens, pregnanediol, total and fractionated 17-oxosteroids, 17-hydroxycorticosteroids and gonadotrophins were measured in preoperative urine samples from fifty nine patients prior to adrenalectomy or hypophysecetomy. These fifty nine patients included thirty six of the original forty one patients, described by HAYWARD et al. (1961). The same trend was observed, namely that the mean 17-OHCS level was higher and the mean aetiocholanolone level was lower in the failure group than in the remission group but the differences between the means were still only marginally significant (P=0.05—0.01) and the overlap between individual values continued to prove so great that the levels of neither hormone could be used alone for the purpose of prediction. When expressed as a simple ratio of 17-OHCS to aetiocholanolone, the difference observed between the success and failure groups could be made more distinct, but the maximum accuracy in prediction, using the urinary hormone levels, was found to result from the calculation of a simple formula, known as a discriminant function.

A discriminant function is a mathematical function of the available measurements that will give the least possible frequency of miscalculation. It is a statistical device, frequently used for agricultural research which, at that time, had not found much favour in medicine.

In this case, the function—calculated by C. C. SPICER—was devised so that when the preoperative urinary levels of the 17-OHCS and aetiocholanolone were substituted in the formula and the result was a positive number, the patient was said to have a positive discriminant and was likely to have a successful response to endocrine ablation. When a negative answer was obtained, the patient was likely to fail to subsequent operation. The formula was:

80—80 (17-OHCS mg per 24 hours)
+ aetiocholanolone μg per 24 hours.

This function discriminated, more exactly than any other mathematical combination of the urinary steroid measurements, between those patients who would benefit and those patients who would fail. SPICER (1966) has since explained in detail the principles that were employed in analysing this particular set of data. The constants on which the discriminant function had been calculated consisted of data from the forty one patients originally described by HAYWARD et al. (1961). Thirty six of these forty one patients were further included in the group of fifty nine patients described by BULBROOK et al. (1960). The remaining twenty three patients in the second study had the discriminant measured before operation but their data were not used in the original calculations of the discriminant. As has

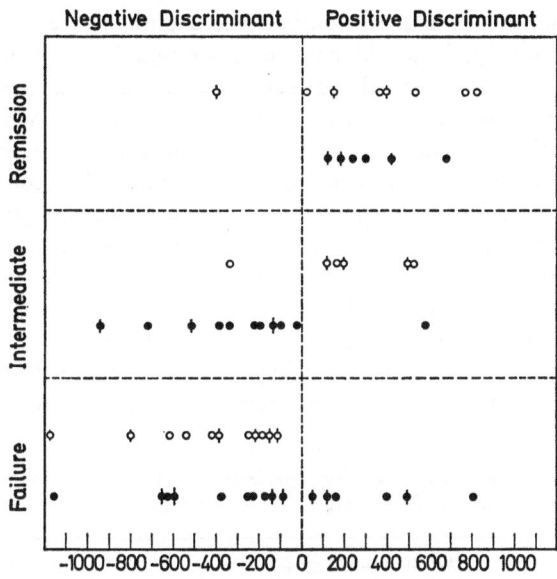

Fig. 7. Correlation between the discriminant and the clinical results of adrenalectomy and hypophysectomy: Clear circles hypophysectomy; black circles adrenalectomy. The discriminant was calculated from data on the cases plotted without vertical lines through the point. Subsequent cases are plotted with vertical lines through the point. (BULBROOK et al., 1960)

already been mentioned, if a sufficient number of substances are measured, it is extremely likely that a statistical correlation with response will be found with one of them. But if this is a chance finding and simply due to the number of different parameters observed, the correlation would tend to disappear when applied to prospective data. Thus the twenty three patients on whom the discriminant was applied, but whose data had not been considered in the calculation of the formula, were a good test of the discriminant's validity.

Fig. 7 shows the correlation between the discriminant function and response in the fifty nine patients. A distinction is made between the thirty six patients used for the original calculation of the discriminant and the twenty three patients who were studied subsequently. It can be seen that, with few exceptions, the original calculations held good for the later cases.

It was also important that the discriminant function should be tested in a prospective trial. This trial had to be designed so that the results would indicate whether the discriminant could be used with reasonable accuracy to select patients for ablation. At that time, ATKINS et al. (1960) had just reported their investigation in which the results of adrenalectomy were compared with those of hypophysectomy; they had shown that hypophysectomy gave marginally better results. It was decided that the discriminant would in future be calculated on all patients to be considered for endocrine ablation. If the discriminant were positive (and hence a good result was expected), the patient would be recommended for hypophysectomy—which ATKINS et al. (1960) had shown to give better results. If the discriminant were negative (indicating a poor response to ablation), it was not felt justified on this basis alone to deny the patient an operation; therefore, these patients had an adrenalectomy, the operation which had previously given slightly poorer results than hypo-physectomy. Theoretically, it would have been preferable to recommend the best operation—hypophysectomy—for all patients, but the facilities were not available to offer this operation to the considerable number of patients who presented for treatment. Some patients would have to be offered adrenalectomy and the selection by means of the discriminant seemed the best compromise. The consequence of this selection would be that if the discriminant was of practical use, the results in the hypophysectomy group would be far better than the results in the adrenalectomy group. The difference in response rate between the groups should be greater than if the operation had been chosen randomly.

ATKINS and his colleagues reported the results of this trial in 1964. Thirty five patients with positive discriminants had a hypophysectomy and thirty three patients with negative discriminants had an adrenalectomy. Table 15 gives a comparison of

Table 15. *Response of patients with positive discriminants subjected to hypophysectomy, and of those with negative discriminants subjected to adrenalectomy.* (ATKINS et al., 1964)

Results	Discriminant — positive (Hypophysectomy)		Discriminant — negative (Adrenalectomy)	
	No.	%	No.	%
Success	16	45.7	3	9.4
Intermediate	8	22.9	7	21.9
Failure	11	31.4	22	68.8
Total	35		32	

X^2 for trend = 12.4, 1 degree of freedom, $P < 0.001$.

the two groups and indicates that the response rate was five times greater in the positive hypophysectomy group than in the negative adrenalectomy group. This difference was highly significant. Comparison of the negative adrenalectomy group with a previous adrenalectomy series, in which the choice of operation had been made by random sample, showed that the discriminant negative adrenalectomies had significantly worse results. On the other hand, comparison of the positive hypo-physectomies with those chosen for the operation by random sample showed that those chosen because of a positive discriminant had a considerably higher response rate, although the difference was not statistically significant.

Although it had been shown that the response rate to adrenalectomy was negli-gible for patients with negative discriminants, it had not been proved that a similar poor response would have resulted if these patients had had a hypophysectomy. A reverse trial was planned in which patients with positive discriminants would have an adrenalectomy and those with negative discriminants a hypophysectomy. It was expected that the former trend would be reversed and that the adrenalectomy results would be much better than those following hypophysectomy. The results of this trial have now been reported (ATKINS et al., 1968 b) and show that the expected reversal has occurred. In table 16, the success rate after adrenalectomy of the patients with positive discriminants is twice as high as the success rate after hypophysectomy of the patients with negative discriminants. This difference is not significant—as was the difference in the opposite direction in the previous trial. It seems that negative hypophysectomies have a better response rate than negative adrenalectomies and possibly positive hypophysectomies have a better response rate than positive adrenalectomies. These results are in accord with those of ATKINS et al. (1960) which showed that in a randomised series, hypophysectomy gave a better response rate and better survival than adrenalectomy.

Table 16. *Response of patients with negative discriminants subjected to adrenalectomy and of those with positive discriminants subjected to hypophysectomy.* (ATKINS et al., 1968)

Results	Discriminant — positive (Adrenalectomy)		Discriminant — negative (Hypophysectomy)	
	No.	%	No.	%
Success	13	(30)	4	(13)
Intermediate	8	(19)	8	(26)
Failure	22	(51)	19	(61)
Total	43		31	

X^2 for trend = 2.0. Not significant.

When a more detailed analysis was carried out on the results of adrenalectomy or hypophysectomy in patients with positive or negative discriminants, a difference in response was observed which depended on whether the patient had had a previous mastectomy. Patients with positive discriminants who had had a hypophysectomy had a response rate of over 40 per cent irrespective of whether a mastectomy had previously been performed. Patients with positive discriminants who had had an adrenalectomy had a response rate of 41 per cent if a previous mastectomy had been carried out but only 11 per cent if the breast had not been removed (ATKINS et al., 1968 a). This unexpected finding may indicate that hormone responsiveness in patients who have advanced tumours when first seen differs from that in patients whose tumours are operable; the success from hypophysectomy in both types of patient suggests a particular dependence on pituitary hormones. Alternatively, the mastectomy itself may affect the endocrine environment; there is certainly evidence that the excretion of metabolites of androgens and corticosteroids is markedly altered for a long time by removal of the breast (BULBROOK and HAYWARD, 1967 b).

Sufficient cases had now been collected to give an estimate of the accuracy of prediction that could be obtained by using the discriminant in practice (HAYWARD and BULBROOK, 1968). To arrive at this estimation, the results which had been used in the original calculation of the discriminant were ignored. Table 17 gives the results in the subsequent 151 patients. The success rate of patients with positive discriminants is more than twice that of patients with negative discriminants; this difference is statistically significant and confirms the validity of the observation on which the discriminant was based.

Nevertheless, from the practical aspect, the accuracy of prediction provided by the discriminant is not good. The success rate of patients with positive discriminants

Table 17. *Response rate from endocrine ablation in patients whose results were not included in the original calculation of the discriminant.* (HAYWARD et al., 1968)

	Discriminant — positive		Discriminant — negative	
	No.	%	No.	%
Success	28	35	11	16
Intermediate	20	25	17	24
Failure	33	41	42	60
Total	81		70	

X^2 for trend $= 7.818$; $p < 0.01$.

Table 18. *The results from endocrine ablation in patients with positive and negative discriminants taking into account the free period and menopausal status.* (HAYWARD and BULBROOK, 1968)

	Discriminant — positive		Discriminant — negative	
	Success	Response rate	Success	Response rate
Either < 2 yrs. free period or < 6 yrs. postmenopausal or both	$22/55$	40%	$3/61$	5%
> 2 yrs. free period > 6 yrs. postmenopausal or premenopausal	$18/50$	36%	$9/42$	21%

is still only 35 per cent, whilst 16 per cent of those with negative discriminants obtain a successful response and would be denied this response if the decision was made not to operate on this group of patients. Some other factors are needed, possibly representing the properties of the tumour itself rather than further measurement of the hormonal environment. As has been shown (see page 54), one property of the tumour that correlates with response to ablation is the free period—this probably giving a measure of the tumour growth rate. Also (see page 55) the relation to the menopause seems to have some predictive value if only to exclude those patients who are in their immediate postmenopausal years. HAYWARD and BULBROOK (1968) reported on the use of the discriminant function for prediction when the free period and the menopausal status were also taken into account. Table 18 shows that the length of the free period and the menopausal status make little difference to the success rate of patients with positive discriminants. Whether these factors are favourable or unfavourable, the response rate is still about 40 per cent. But those patients with negative discriminants, who also have a free period of less than two years or are within six years of the menopause, have a response rate from adrenalectomy or hypophysectomy of only five per cent. This is a large group, representing nearly one third of the patients presenting for ablation and, on the basis of these figures, HAYWARD and BULBROOK (1968) suggest that these patients should not be operated on. The remainder of the discriminant negative group (i. e. those who have a free period of more than two years or who are not within six years of the menopause) have a response rate of 16 per cent which many physicians would consider high enough for an operation to be recommended.

The discriminant function can be a practical aid in the management of advanced breast cancer by helping a surgeon to reject with confidence approximately one third of those patients whom he would consider for a major ablative procedure. At least, he will be able to do this if the hormone determinations, on which the discriminant function is based, are readily available to him. Unfortunately this is seldom the case. The estimations—particularly the assay of aetiocholanolone—are complicated and seldom within the compass of the routine pathological laboratory. Aetiocholanolone is one of the three urinary androgen metabolites which form the 11-deoxy-17-oxosteroids. The levels of the other two members of this group (androsterone and dehydroepiandrosterone) vary directly with the level of aetiocholanolone but were not included in the original calculation of the discriminant because the best correlation with response had been obtained by using aetiocholanolone alone. Very probably if either of the others had been used, almost exactly the same results would have been obtained. The determination of the total 11-deoxy-17-oxosteroids, representing the combined levels of aetiocholanolone, androsterone and dehydroepiandrosterone, is a relatively simple estimation and does not involve very complicated techniques. MILLER et al. (1967) measured the 17-OHCS, the total 11-deoxy-17-oxosteroids and aetiocholanolone, in a series of breast cancer patients and controls. They then expressed the levels of the 11-deoxy-17-oxosteroids and the 17-OHCS as a ratio, and in each patient compared the value of this ratio with the discriminant. They found that the ratio varied directly with the discriminant. Almost all the patients who had a ratio above 0.16 had a positive discriminant, whilst those whose ratio was below 0.13 had a negative discriminant. Subsequently, THOMAS, BULBROOK and HAYWARD (1967) calculated the ratio of the 11-deoxy-17-oxosteroids to the 17-OHCS in their patients who had previously had an adrenalectomy or hypophysectomy and compared it with the value of the discriminant. They found that those patients who had a ratio above 0.17 had a success rate almost identical with those who had a positive discriminant. Similarly, those patients who had a ratio equal to or below 0.17 had a success rate the same as those with a negative discriminant. This ratio may give similar results to those obtained with the original discriminant and, with its ease of calculation, may prove more useful in practice.

Other workers have also shown that measurements of steroid excretion correlate with the response to endocrine ablation. JURET, HAYEM and FLEISLER (1964) found that the combined amounts of urinary aetiocholanolone and androsterone varied directly with the response of their patients to pituitary ablation by 90 Yttrium. When the sum of these compounds was over 2.0 mg per 24 hours, they observed a 70 per cent success rate, whereas when the level was below 0.3 mg per 24 hours, only 7 per cent responded. Independently, in Japan, KUMAOKA et al. (1968) were able to correlate the preoperative urinary levels of the 11-deoxy-17-oxosteroids with response to bilateral adrenalectomy. Normal levels were associated with favourable results and low levels with failure. Also FOTHERBY et al. (1968) have measured the discriminant function and the ratio of the 17-oxogenic steroids to the combined excretion of androsterone and aetiocholanolone in patients before pituitary ablation or additive therapy. Their preliminary results have shown that both the discriminant function and the ratio correlate with the response to treatment.

Other discriminants have also been proposed. WILSON and MOORE (1968) have calculated a discriminant function, based on the incremental ratios of the 17-OHCS and 17-oxosteroids, and the free interval. The incremental ratios are calculated from the response of the adrenal to stimulation by ACTH. They believe that this measure of the adrenal potential gives more valuable information than the measurements of the urinary androgen metabolites from the unstimulated adrenal. Using their discriminant, they were able to select 80 per cent of the patients who responded and 75 per cent of those who did not respond in a retrospective series of 100 adrenal-ectomies.

More accurate prediction is still needed and can probably be obtained. It may be that more factors should be taken into consideration and more complicated discriminants formulated. The application of the measurements that are now being carried out is largely empirical and little is known of the physiological meaning of the discriminant. Investigation of the metabolic pathway of androgen or corticoid synthesis and breakdown is complicated. Accurate methods do not exist for measuring the secretion rates of many of the compounds and little work has been done to investigate the disturbance of steroid metabolism that seems to be present in many patients with breast cancer. Recently, DESHPANDE and his colleagues (1967) investigated adrenal steroid biogenesis in patients with advanced breast cancer. In nine patients undergoing adrenalectomy, one adrenal was perfused with tritiated Δ^5 pregnenolone. The conversion of this compound to dehydroepiandrosterone (DHA) and cortisol was then estimated from serial samples of adrenal venous blood. The discriminant function was also measured on a preoperative urine sample.

The results showed a positive correlation between the ratio of adrenal biosynthesis of DNA and cortisol and the discriminant function. The patients with a negative discriminant, and hence with a poor prognosis following adrenalectomy, seemed less able to convert pregnenolone to DNA. DESHPANDE and his colleagues suggested that this might be due to a deficiency in the 17-desmolase enzyme system, responsible for the cleavage of the C_{21} side chain.

Summary and Conclusions

1. The microscopical features of a tumour give no guide to response to adrenalectomy or hypophysectomy but the site of metastases affects remission. Visceral metastases probably herald the worst prognosis but patients should not be refused ablation on these grounds alone.

2. A successful response to previous castration may indicate a successful response to ablation but response to previous hormone therapy gives no guide.

3. Patients who are within 6 years of the menopause or who have a free period of less than 2 years tend to do badly.

4. Pre-operative urinary oestrogen levels do not correlate with response. Continued oestrogen excretion after ablation is not necessarily associated with failure.

5. Pre-operative urinary androgen and corticosteroid levels correlate with response. When the hormone levels are combined in a discriminant function, and taking the free period and menopausal status into account, a moderately accurate forecast can be made.

6. The use of the discriminant function, or of a simple ratio of the 11-deoxy-17-oxo-steroids to the 17-OHCS, enables patients to be identified who will stand a less than 5 per cent chance of responding to adrenalectomy or hypophysectomy. This group represents nearly one third of the patients considered for ablative procedures.

References

ALLEN, B. J., HAYWARD, J. L., MERIVALE, W. H. H.: The excretion of 17-ketosteroids in the urine of patients with generalised carcinomatosis secondary to carcinoma of the breast. Lancet **1957 I**, 496.

APPLEBY, J. I., GIBSON, G., NORYMBERSKI, J. K., STUBBS, R. D.: Indirect analysis of corticosteroids. I. The determination of 17-hydroxy-corticosteroids. Biochem. J. **60**, 453 (1955).

ATKINS, H. J. B., BULBROOK, R. D., FALCONER, M. A., HAYWARD, J. L., MacLEAN, K. S., SCHURR, P. H.: Urinary steroid estimations in the prediction of response to adrenalectomy or hypophysectomy. Lancet **1964 II**, 1133.

— — — — — — Ten years experience of steroid assays in the management of breast cancer. Lancet **1968 a II**, 1255.

— — — — — — Urinary steroids in the prediction of response to adrenalectomy or hypophysectomy. A second clinical trial. Lancet **1968b II**, 1261.

— FALCONER, M. A., HAYWARD, J. L., MacLEAN, K. S., SCHURR, P. H.: The timing of adrenalectomy and of hypophysectomy in the treatment of advanced breast cancer. Lancet **1966 I**, 827.

— — — — — ARMITAGE, P.: Adrenalectomy and hypophysectomy for advanced cancer of the breast. Lancet **1960 I**, 1148.

BAULD, W. S.: A method for the determination of oestriol, oestrone, and oestradiol-17β in human urine by partition chromatography and colorimetric estimation. Biochem. J. **63**, 483 (1956).

BECK, J. C., BLAIR, A. J., GRIFFITHS, M. M., ROSENFELD, M. W., McGARRY, E. E.: In search or hormonal factors as an aid in predicting the outcome of breast carcinoma. In: Proc. Sixth Canadian Cancer Conference. Pergamon Press 1966, p. 3.

BLOCK, G. E., VIAL, A. B., McCARTHY, J. D., PORTER, C. W., COLLER, F. A.: Adrenalectomy in advanced mammary cancer. Surg. Gynec. Obstet. **108**, 651 (1959).

BROWN, J. B.: A chemical method for the determination of oestriol, oestrone and oestradiol in human urine. Biochem. J. **60**, 185 (1955).

— BULBROOK, R. D., GREENWOOD, F. C.: An additional purification step for a method for estimating oestriol, oestrone and oestradiol 17β in human urine. J. Endocr. **16**, 49 (1957).

— FALCONER, C. W. A., STRONG, J. A.: Urinary oestrogens of adrenal origin in women with breast cancer. J. Endocr. **19**, 52 (1959).

BULBROOK, R. D.: Hormone assays in human breast cancer. Vitam. and Horm. **23**, 329 (1965).

— GREENWOOD, F. C., HADFIELD, G. J., SCOWEN, E. F.: Adrenalectomy in breast cancer. An attempt to correlate clinical results with oestrogen production. Brit. med. J. **1958a I**, 12.

— — — — Hypophysectomy in breast cancer. An attempt to correlate clinical results with oestrogen production. Brit. med. J. **1958 b I**, 15.

— — HAYWARD, J. L.: Selection of breast cancer patients for adrenalectomy or hypophysectomy by determination of urinary 17-hydroxycorticosteroids and aetiocholanolone. Lancet **1960 I**, 1154.

— — Factors influencing the prognostic value of urinary steroid determinations. In: Major Endocrine Surgery for the Treatment of Cancer of the Breast in Advanced Stages. Eds.: M. DARGENT and CL. ROMIEU. Lyon: Simep Editions 1967, p. 37.

DAO, T. L., NEMOTO, T.: An evaluation of adrenalectomy and androgen in disseminated mammary carcinoma. Surg. Gynec. Obstet. **121**, 1257 (1965).

DESHPANDE, N., JENSEN, V., BULBROOK, R. D., DOOUSS, T. W.: In vivo steroidogenesis by the human adrenal gland. Steroids **9**, 393 (1967).

FAIRGRIEVE, J.: Selective criteria for surgical removal of the endocrine glands in advanced breast cancer. Surg. Gynec. Obstet. **120**, 371 (1965).

FOTHERBY, K., SELLWOOD, R. A., BURN, J. I.: Urinary steroid excretion in patients with advanced breast cancer. Brit. J. Surg. **55**, 868 (1968).

HAYWARD, J. L., BULBROOK, R. D.: Urinary steroids and prognosis in breast cancer. In: Prognostic Factors in Breast Cancer. Eds.: A. P. M. FORREST and P. B. KUNKLER. Edinburgh: Livingstone 1968, p. 383.

HAYWARD, J. L., BULBROOK, R. D., GREENWOOD, F. C.: Hormone assays and prognosis in breast cancer. Med. Soc. Endocrin. 10, 144 (1961).

HOBKIRK, R., FORREST, A. P. M.: Urinary steroid patterns in breast cancer. Lancet 1957 I, 636.

HUGGINS, C., DAO, T. L.-Y.: Characteristics of adrenal-dependent mammary cancers. Ann. Surg. 140, 497 (1954).

JURET, P., HAYEM, M., FLEISLER, A.: A propos de 150 implantations d'yttrium radio-actif intra-hypophysaires dans la traitement du cancer du sein a une étade avancée. J. Chir. (Paris) 87, 409 (1964).

KELLIE, A. E., WADE, A. P.: The analysis of urinary 17-oxosteroids by gradient elution. Biochem. J. 66, 196 (1957).

KLOPPER, A., MICHIE, E. A., BROWN, J. B.: A method for the determination of urinary pregnanediol. J. Endocr. 12, 209 (1955).

KUMAOKA, S., SAKAUCHI, N., ABE, O., KUSAMA, M., TAKATANI, O.: Urinary 17-ketosteroid excretion of women with advanced breast cancer. J. Clin. Endocr. 28, 667 (1968).

LIPSETT, M. B., WHITMORE, W. F., TREVES, N., WEST, C. D., RANDALL, H. T., PEARSON, O. F.: Bilateral adrenalectomy in the palliation of metastatic breast cancer. Cancer 10, 111 (1957).

LORAINE, J. A., BROWN, J. B.: A method for the quantitative determination of gonado-trophins in the urine of non-pregnant human subjects. J. Endocr. 18, 77 (1959).

MACDONALD, I.: Endocrine ablation in disseminated mammary carcinoma. Surg. Gynec. Obstet. 115, 215 (1962).

McCALISTER, A., WELBOURN, R. B., EDELSTYN, G. J. A., LYONS, A. R., TAYLOR, A. R., GLEADHILL, C. A., GORDON D. S., COLE, J. O. Y.: Factors influencing response to hypo-physectomy for advanced cancer of the breast. Brit. med. J. 1961 I, 613.

MILLER, M., DURANT, J. A., JACOBS, A. G., ALLISON, JACQUELINE F.: Alternative discriminat-ing function for determining hormone dependency of breast cancer. Brit. med. J. 1967 I, 147.

PEARSON, O. H., RAY, B. S.: Hypophysectomy in the treatment of metastatic mammary cancer. Am. J. Surg. 99, 544 (1960).

PLANTIN, L. O., BIRKE, G., DISZFALUSY, E., FRANKSON, C., HELLSTROM, J., HULTBERG, S., WESTMAN, A.: On the excretion pattern by 17-oxosteroids and corticosteroids in breast cancer. In: Endocrine Aspects of Breast Cancer. Ed.: A. R. CURRIE. Edinburgh-London: Livingstone 1958, p. 224.

SPICER, C. C.: Inter-relation of methods of assessment: statistical problems and techniques. In: Clinical Evaluation in Breast Cancer. Eds.: J. L. HAYWARD and R. D. BULBROOK. London-New York: Academic Press 1966, p. 231.

THOMAS, B. S., BULBROOK, R. D., HAYWARD, J. L.: Urinary steroid assays and response to endocrine ablation. Brit. med. J. 3, 523 (1967).

WILSON, R. E., MOORE, F. D.: Biochemical and clinical factors in the selection of patients for endocrine surgery. In: Prognostic Factors in Breast Cancer. Eds.: A. P. M. FORREST and P. B. KUNKLER. Edinburgh: Livingstone 1968, p. 399.

WOLFF, B.: The differential cell count in cancer of the breast and response to hormone therapy. Guy's Hosp. Rep. 106, 53 (1957).

Chapter 5

Androgens and Oestrogens

The use of sex hormones for the treatment of breast cancer probably contributed more to the management of the advanced disease than the advent of any other therapy. Their value in patients too ill for more severe treatment, their relative lack of debilitating side effects, and the long periods of remission that may be obtained, combine to give hormones a measure of advantage over any other therapy. But it is this very simplicity of use which has resulted in a relative lack of endeavour by clinical research workers to investigate their mode of action. There is little encouragement to investigate the features which might predict those patients who may benefit from hormone therapy when it is so easy to try the drugs clinically on all cases. Androgens or oestrogens can be administered without the patient being admitted to hospital, and the response of the tumour soon provides the answer as to whether or not the treatment will work.

Nor have the results of research so far attempted been of much practical help to the clinician. The same or similar compounds are used now as were used twenty years ago with the same degree of success. In spite of the length of time (nearly three decades) during which hormone therapy has been available, there is still little knowledge of the mode of action. Two groups of hormones—androgens and oestrogens—with dissimilar physiological properties, appear to have nearly the same clinical effect and it is not known how either of them work.

1. Response

a) Success Rate

The assessment of response to hormone therapy present many of the difficulties described in the section dealing with response to ovarian ablation. Before a true estimate can be made of the response rate of patients receiving androgens or oestrogens, there must be agreement on the precise criteria to be used in deciding whether a treatment has been successful.

Many series have been reported (see for instance CUTLER and SCHLEMENSON, 1948; GALTON, 1950; DOUGLAS, 1952; SEGALOFF et al., 1953; FOSS, 1956; GOLDENBERG, 1964) and there have also been several reviews (see LEWISON and TRIMBLE, 1956; KENNEDY, 1965). But the protocols for assessing response have differed so widely that it is difficult to interpret the results, and certainly no valid comparison can be made between the various series or compounds used.

On the other hand, some of the investigations on the effects of androgens and oestrogens has been done within series rather than in comparison with other series.

If done within series, the precise definition of success is not quite so important, providing it is constant and not liable to misinterpretation or bias by the observer.

For instance, the Sub-Committee on Breast and Genital Cancer of the American Medical Association (1960) conducted a retrospective enquiry into the effect of oestrogen or androgen administration in 1,983 patients with advanced breast cancer. Rules were formulated which laid down the essential information required about a patient before she could be included in the study. Many patients were rejected, either because data on response or follow-up were incomplete or because the treatment had been inadequate. Nine hundred and forty-four of the original patients were finally considered suitable for analysis. To assess response, a protocol was used which demanded that one or more dominant metastasis must undergo a distinct measurable decrease in size without progression in any other lesion—although no restriction was placed on the time this remission had to last. On this basis, the response rate in 580 patients on androgen therapy was 21.4 per cent and in 346 patients on oestrogen therapy 36.8 per cent.

There are two points arising from these results. Firstly no attempt was made to compare these response rates with those reported by other investigators and from other centres. The reader has to interpret the results in the light of the criteria of response on which they have been judged. Thus no claim is made for a response rate from androgen therapy, but rather for a response rate observed with this particular interpretation of remission. Secondly, and as a consequence, although the response rates may have limited meaning by themselves, they have considerable meaning when they are compared one with another. The figures of 21.4 per cent and 36.8 per cent have been obtained by the same investigators applying the same set of rules on patients chosen in the same way. A direct comparison is possible and the results may be meaningful.

Nowadays, this type of retrospective enquiry is sometimes derided. It is felt that without the strictures of a controlled clinical trial, investigations can have little meaning. CUTLER (1966) has recently answered this criticism and emphasised some of the very real advantages that can result from a retrospective enquiry. Nevertheless, data obtained under these conditions are highly selected (in the American Medical Association enquiry, over 1,000 patients were discarded to accept 944) and, however careful the selectors may be and whatever pains may be taken to eliminate bias, this degree of selection carries with it many dangers.

Suffice it to say therefore that an expression of the success rate following hormone therapy can have little meaning until there is agreement on the criteria of response. At the present, the only acceptable figures are those comparing response to androgens with response to oestrogens within one series.

b) Survival

Some of our knowledge of the action of administered hormones has resulted from controlled clinical trials. But there have been far more reports of uncontrolled series and many of these have provided useful information. A constant finding is that patients responding to oestrogen or androgen therapy live longer than those who do not respond. (Co-operative Breast Cancer Group, 1964 a and b, Council on Drugs, American Medical Association 1960.) This does not necessarily mean that a patient's life span is increased if she has a favourable response to hormone therapy.

There may be two types of breast cancer; in one type, the patient has a naturally long survival and responds to hormone therapy; in the other there is a naturally short survival and her disease fails to respond. On the other hand, it has been shown (Council on Drugs, American Medical Association 1960) in a comparable series that although patients not responding to androgens or oestrogens survive a very similar length of time (ten and eleven months respectively), those responding to oestrogens live considerably longer than those responding to androgens (twenty seven months compared with twenty months). This can only result, either from oestrogen therapy increasing the survival rate, or from androgen therapy decreasing it.

On the evidence, it seems likely that successful hormone therapy slightly increases the length of survival. Confirmation of this could come only from a controlled clinical trial comparing hormone therapy with the administration of a placebo.

c) Histological Changes

Little is known of the progressive histological changes that may occur following hormone therapy. A tumour mass would have to be sectioned at weekly or monthly intervals to obtain a meaningful histological pattern of the progress of remission. This would be difficult to justify ethically, but some idea of the changes can be obtained by sequential removal of skin nodules.

An American Medical Association report (1951) likened the effect of successful hormone therapy on malignant tissue to that produced by ionising radiation. In some instances, there was complete disappearance of the tumour tissue contained in skin nodules and breast deposits. But the effect was not constant. Sometimes, whilst a proportion of the tumour tissue was completely destroyed, there were cells which were damaged but could recover and also cells which seemed unaffected. GOWING (1966) has recently summarised these effects in describing the results of radiation therapy on tumour cells, stroma and the surrounding normal tissue. KOLLER (1944) was able to examine serial biopsy sections from a tumour that was treated successfully by stilboestrol. He described initial nuclear vacuolation, cytoplasmic hyperchromism and a reduction in the mitotic count. In subsequent sections, the mitotic rate increased but with a marked number of abnormal divisions.

EMERSON et al. (1953) studied the tumours of 14 patients who were receiving oestrogens for advanced breast cancer. All the tumours were in regression and they remarked on the degeneration of the cells and the surrounding cicatrization. However, they also noted that malignant cells survived even in complete regression and were presumably the source of subsequent tumour growth.

WOLFF (1957) carried out differential cell counts on biopsies taken from fifteen women with advanced breast cancer. These women were then given oestrogen therapy and a further biopsy was taken of a skin nodule. In ten out of the fifteen cases, the cell counts of the biopsy taken after oestrogen treatment, showed a decrease in the percentage of mitotic cells and a corresponding increase in the percentage of resting cells.

2. Factors Associated with Hormone Action

Many attempts have been made to correlate the response to hormone therapy with identifiable features of the patient or of the tumour under treatment. These have met with varied degrees of success and, although some associations have been found, it is doubtful whether these have contributed much either to the understanding of the mechanisms involved or to the management of the disease. Also, many of the reports are unconfirmed or conflicting.

a) Age

There is a positive association between response to hormone therapy and age. An old patient stands more chance of a remission than a young one. The American Medical Association report (1960) showed that the pre- and immediate postmenopausal remission rates following androgen therapy were almost the same (20.0 per cent and 21.9 per cent). But after the menopause, the remission rate increased with advancing age. Similarly, the Co-operative Breast Cancer Group (1964 b) showed that the highest percentage of remissions following testosterone therapy occurred in patients who were more than ten years postmenopausal. The lowest remission rate occurred in patients who were less than one year postmenopausal.

The same phenomenon has been observed following oestrogen therapy. HAYWARD (1957) reported on the remission experience of ninety two patients with advanced breast cancer who had been treated with stilboestrol. To estimate response he used both the Mean Clinical Value (see pp. 34—35) and the success rate. HAYWARD's patients were divided into three groups according to age:

1. Those under 55
2. Those aged from 55—69
3. Those aged 70 and over.

Using the Mean Clinical Value, a comparison of response at six and twelve months after the commencement of oestrogen treatment revealed that patients over seventy had a significantly better remission than patients between fifty-five and sixty-nine, and that patients between fifty-five and sixty-nine had a significantly better remission rate than patients under fifty-five. Using the success rate to express response, it was shown that 60 per cent of patients over seventy benefitted from oestrogen therapy, compared with 40 per cent of those between fifty-five and sixty-nine and 18 per cent of those under fifty-five.

b) The Site of Metastases

It is generally believed that metastases at certain sites have identifiable behavioural characteristics. This would seem a logical consequence of the observation that metastatic spread from breast cancer follows one of several distinct patterns. Thus the disease may spread locally with few, if any, distant deposits; alternatively, there may be no local spread but widespread skeletal deposits; or occasionally visceral deposits may be dominant. Sometimes the pattern may be mixed, but usually one or other system seems to be involved to the relative exclusion of the others. The likely reason for this is that the metabolism of tumour tissue differs from one growth to another; in one case, blood born tumour cells may find that bone provides a suitable medium for growth; in another case, only the liver may provide a suitable environment. If small alterations in tumour metabolism can cause such major differences in the spread of the disease, then it is not unreasonable to suggest that the same or similar alterations in metabolism might determine the response of the tumour to hormone therapy. Thus, the type of cell which finds bone a suitable environment for growth might also be the type that is sensitive to a particular hormone.

There is little agreement between investigators either on whether metastases at different sites respond in the same way or, if they are reported to respond differently, on which metastases respond most favourably. The American Medical Association report (1960) was unable to demonstrate any difference in response for metastases at different sites. HAYWARD (1957) found that patients with metastases in the liver fared worse following oestrogen therapy and patients with bony deposits fared best, but the differences were not significant. GOLDENBERG, BAILAR and LOWRY (1964), in a report on the survival of women with hormone treated breast cancer, found that patients with osseous and local disease enjoyed a longer survival than those with visceral disease. The Co-operative Breast Cancer Group, in their various publications, have always gone to great pains to sub-group their patients receiving hormone therapy according to the dominant lesion. They have written into their protocol (SEGALOFF, 1966) a code for deciding which lesion is dominant in any patient. In a review of testosterone propionate therapy in breast cancer (Co-operative Breast Cancer Group, 1964 b), they found that most remissions (31.5 per cent) occurred in patients with soft tissue metastases (breast, skin or gland). Patients with bony or visceral metastases had the same response rate (18 per cent) which was significantly worse than the patients with soft tissue metastases; they were unable to demonstrate any difference in survival rate between the three groups.

The only constant finding seems to be that patients with visceral metastases (principally lung, liver and brain) have a lower incidence of remission and possibly a worse survival than patients with metastases at other sites. It is not known whether this is due to inherent differences in the hormone responsiveness of this type of metastasis or whether it is a result of the location of the diseased tissue. Large areas of neoplastic tissue in a vital organ such as the liver or in the lungs must present a greater threat to the host than secondaries in skin or lymph nodes. Similarly, if secondaries in the brain improve, there can be no subsequent regeneration of the brain tissue and it may be difficult to prove that a remission has occurred.

c) Host Factors

The interval between the primary operation for early breast cancer (e. g. mastectomy) and recurrence is called the free period or free interval. The free period may give information not only on the natural growth rate of the tumour but also on its hormone responsiveness. For instance, the length of the free period correlates with the subsequent response to endocrine ablation. A free period of over two years indicates that a good response is likely from adrenalectomy of hypophysectomy, whereas a free period of less than two years heralds a poor response (see page 54). There is some evidence that a similar correlation exists between the free period and the response to hormones by administration. In patients receiving hormone therapy, GOLDENBERG et al. (1964) were able to demonstrate a direct correlation between the free period and survival after the first detection of recurrence or metastasis. Their definition of hormone therapy included castration, administration of androgens, oestrogens, progestogens or corticoids as well as adrenalectomy or hypophysectomy and it is not clear which was the predominant treatment; most of their patients had more than one of the options. When the free period was less than one year, 35 per cent survived more than two years after recurrence; when the free period was five years or more, 65 per cent survived more than two years. They believed that the importance of the free period was such that it tended to over-ride other factors affecting response such as age or tumour size. The American Medical Association report (1960) also demonstrated a significant correlation between the free period and both the incidence of regression and the survival after hormone therapy.

HAYWARD (1957) investigated the effect of parity on hormone response; he divided his patients into two groups; parous and nulliparous. The thirty-two nulliparous patients appeared to derive much greater benefit from oestrogen therapy than the fifty-two patients who had borne children. This difference was shown to be significant. In his series, the incidence of side effects from oestrogen therapy (nipple pigmentation, nausea and vomiting, bleeding per vaginam) did not correlate with response.

d) The Primary Complex

There is little evidence that features of the original breast tumour and axillary nodes are associated with response to subsequent hormone therapy.

The report of the American Medical Association (1960) noted that older postmenopausal patients had an increased remission rate only if a radical mastectomy had originally been performed. On the other hand, HAYWARD (1957), although also demonstrating an increased rate of remission in old people given oestrogen therapy, was unable to show any difference in response according to whether or not the primary had been removed.

GOLDENBERG et al. (1964) analysed their results of hormone therapy to see whether the size of the primary tumour was correlated with survival after recurrence. They were able to show that patients with small primary tumours survived longer than those with large tumours, although this observation may have little to do with response to hormone therapy. CUTLER (1966) has described an investigation by ZIPPIN in which a direct correlation was demonstrated between tumour size and survival after mastectomy irrespective of whether the patients had received hormones when the disease became advanced. GOLDENBERG and his colleagues also investigated the effect on survival of the situation of the primary within the breast and of the degree of axillary node involvement, but were unable to demonstrate any association. Also, the local characteristics of the primary tumour (e. g. Muscle fixation, skin involvement, etc.) did not correlate with survival after recurrence.

e) The Histology of the Tumour

One supposition has been that if the tumour was highly differentiated there would be more likelihood of it responding to hormone administration. Each patient in the American Medical Association report (1960) had the diagnosis of breast cancer confirmed histologically. The histology of the primary tumour was also compared with the response to hormone therapy but no correlation between tumour differentiation and hormone response could be demonstrated. WOLFF (1957) studied the differential cell count in tumour biopsy specimens taken from fifty-nine patients to be treated with oestrogens. She reported that the majority of patients who had a good subsequent response to oestrogen therapy had an initial resting cell count of over 97 per cent and a mitotic cell count of under 2 per cent. She suggested that high resting cell and low mitotic cell counts tended to be related to successful treatment, but that the individual values were not sufficiently consistent to be used as indications for such treatment.

HAYWARD (1957) was unable to correlate the Grade of the primary lesion with response to subsequent hormone therapy.

3. Choice of Compound and Dosage

Much of the research effort into hormone therapy—particularly in the U.S.A.—has been aimed at finding the best compounds for therapeutic use. Ideally, these compounds should have the maximum effect on the tumour, produce remissions in as many patients as possible and have the minimum side effects.

The Co-operative Breast Cancer Group has spent many years in attempts to produce and evaluate new hormones for the treatment of advanced breast cancer. The evaluation of the new compounds is made by comparing their clinical effects with those of reference compounds. These reference compounds are hormones of known effect such as testosterone propionate. Each new compound is tested against the reference compound in a clinical trial. Ideally, the investigator in these trials does not know which of his patients is receiving the new compound and which the reference compound—although this is not always possible. Before the code is broken, his results are analysed retrospectively by a panel of assessors. Their judgement of the success or failure of treatment is based on an appraisal of the serial measurements of lesions, of serial photographs of visible lesions and, where appropriate, of serial x-rays. A very strict protocol is used so that rigid rules govern the inclusion of a patient in the trial and the final assessment of the results of the treatment (SEGALOFF, 1966). Several clinicians may investigate the same drug and usually forty to fifty patients are used in each investigation, half receiving the compound under test and half receiving the reference compound.

Most of the compounds tested have been androgens, although oestrogens have been compared with androgens in some of the studies. In spite of the wealth of new and apparently promising compounds that have been studied and in spite of the complex and nearly foolproof methods used for assessment, the results of this work have been disappointing. Some new androgens, such as fluoxymesterone and possibly Δ_1 testololactone (SEGALOFF et al., 1960, 1962; CANTINO and GORDAN, 1962), have been shown to have as good a clinical effect as testosterone propionate, whilst having less side effects. But no new drug has yet been produced which consistently gives a better incidence of clinical remission. Testosterone propionate as a reference compound has always proved the equal of the drug under test. Also, in spite of the strict protocol, there has been remarkable variation in the remission rates obtained by different observers, and even for the same drug by the same observer on different occasions.

The conclusion seems to be that there is a fixed maximum remission rate that can be obtained by androgen therapy. This remission rate is a constant and is a feature of the number of responsive tumours in a population. It is not increased by minor alterations in the chemical structure of the drugs used for treatment. If the tumour is unresponsive, no androgen will have an effect; if the tumour is responsive, most androgens act equally and the only helpful effect of structural alterations to the androgen molecule is to inhibit side effects.

Most androgens have both an anabolising and a masculinising effect. The ideal compound would seem to be one which has the minimum virilising effect, whilst retaining sufficient properties as an androgen to produce a remission. Many such compounds are now available and some of these have been further developed so that their action after a single dose may last days or even weeks. Nandrolone phenyl propionate (Durabolin) need only be given by intramuscular injection once a week and 19-nor-androstanolone decanoate (Decadurabolin) need only be given once every three weeks. Both compounds have an anabolic and anti-tumour effect, whilst not giving rise to virilisation in more than about 10 per cent of patients. There are many other similar compounds now available, some given by intramuscular injection and some given orally.

Far less work has been done on the development of new oestrogens; this is particularly remarkable considering that oestrogens are superior to androgens in the treatment of breast cancer in postmenopausal women (see page 77). However, the mechanism of tumour response observed for androgens probably holds good for oestrogens. Either a tumour will respond to oestrogen therapy—and it will not make much difference which kind of synthetic oestrogen is used—or it will not respond. In the latter case, no alteration to the oestrogen molecule will increase its effect on the tumour. Side effects are not such a problem with oestrogen therapy and, probably for this reason, little work has been done to produce a compound that the patient will tolerate better. Stilboestrol and ethinyl oestradiol are the drugs most commonly used and, although patients occasionally may complain of nausea or vomiting, one or other of the compounds is usually well tolerated.

For many of the commonly administered hormones, the dose and frequency of administration which will give an optimum tumour response is not known. Presumably, very small amounts have no physiological effect whereas very large amounts are unnecessary. But the question remains whether variation of dosage within the usual therapeutic range affects remission.

Animal work indicates that androgens and oestrogens may have different and distinctive dosage response curves (SEGALOFF, 1966). In particular, small doses of oestrogens may stimulate a tumour to grow whilst large doses inhibit growth. This phenomenon is not confined to animals and can also be observed when treating patients with breast cancer. Small doses of stilboestrol can increase tumour growth rate and relatively large amounts are required to attain a remission. The optimum dosage is not known. Five milligrams of stilboestrol daily is almost certainly too small; probably fifteen milligrams daily is sufficient but a dose of fifty milligrams daily is safest. This is usually well tolerated but, if side effects (particularly nausea and vomiting) are severe, ethinyl oestradiol one milligram daily can be substituted.

There is less information on response following various doses of androgens. In animal studies, very small amounts of some compounds may stimulate the tumour and in other instances large doses may have the same effect (SEGALOFF, 1966). Clinically, the accepted dose depends on the androgen used. Of those compounds commonly employed, fifty milligrams weekly of nandrolone phenyl propionate, one-hundred milligrams thrice weekly of testosterone propionate, or twenty milligrams daily of fluoxymesterone (Ultandren) would be effective amounts.

There is a great need for accurate dosage response curves to be calculated for the hormones commonly used in the treatment of human breast cancer. Possibly tumours with different metabolic patterns would also respond differently to various doses of the same hormone. Current work in progress investigating the response of human tumours to hormones in various doses may throw some light on this problem in the near future.

4. Comparison of Androgens and Oestrogens

Many studies, both retrospective and prospective, have been carried out on the relative merits of androgens and oestrogens. From these studies, two conclusions are constantly reported.

1. In almost all postmenopausal age groups, oestrogens give a better response rate than androgens.

2. The response rate from both groups of compounds increases with advancing age.

The American Medical Association report (1960) reviewed and compared the action of androgens and oestrogens in 944 patients. When other factors had been taken into account, it was concluded that oestrogens gave a higher response rate than androgens at all ages after the fourth postmenopausal year (21 per cent for androgens, 35 per cent for oestrogens). However, this difference was only significant over the age of seventy. During the four years following the menopause, the incidence of remission following androgen or oestrogen therapy was found to be similar.

There were few data on the effect of oestrogens before the menopause because most observers believed that acceleration of tumour growth could occur (NATHANSON, 1950) and the drug was seldom used. In fact, there is little direct evidence for this but more information would come only from a prospective trial which would be difficult to justify. At the present, in premenopausal breast cancer patients, it would seem prudent to withold oestrogens as therapy both for the disease and for other unrelated conditions. In particular, oestrogens should not be given to treat menopausal symptoms nor, in association with progestogens, be used for contraceptive purposes.

No difference was found in the incidence of response following androgen therapy or oestrogen therapy in patients with visceral or bony deposits—this was an unexpected finding because androgens are generally believed to be the treatment of choice for patients with skeletal deposits. In patients with soft tissue lesions (breast, skin and gland), oestrogens appear to give a significantly better response rate.

KENNEDY (1965) described a comparison of stilboestrol and testosterone therapy in advanced breast cancer. Unlike the American Medical Association (1960) report, KENNEDY's study was a randomised controlled trial, using the protocol of the Co-operative Breast Cancer Group (SEGALOFF, 1966). He compared the response rate of fifty nine patients, receiving testosterone propionate, with that of fifty five patients receiving stilboestrol. Tables 19 and 20 give the incidence of objective remission in each group; the total remission rate for patients receiving stilboestrol was significantly better than the total remission rate for the patients receiving testosterone propionate. Details are also given in Tables 19 and 20 of the remission experience when the patients were subgrouped according to the dominant lesion. KENNEDY

Table 19. *Incidence of remission in patients receiving testosterone propionate, expressed as number of objective remissions / total number of patients treated.* (KENNEDY, 1965)

Dominant lesion	Postmenopausal age in years				Total	Per cent
	< 1	1—5	5—10	10+		
Breast	$0/2$	$0/4$	$1/1$	$1/5$	$2/12$	16.7
Osseous	$0/2$	$0/4$	$1/2$	$1/7$	$2/15$	13.3
Visceral	$0/3$	$0/7$	$0/4$	$2/18$	$2/32$	6.2
Total	$0/7$	$0/15$	$2/7$	$4/30$	$6/59$	10.1

Table 20. *Incidence of remission in patients receiving stilboestrol, expressed as number of objective remissions / total number of patients treated.* (KENNEDY, 1965)

Dominant lesion	Postmenopausal age in years				Total	Per cent
	< 1	1—5	5—10	10+		
Breast	$0/1$	$0/2$	$1/2$	$5/11$	$6/16$	37.5
Osseous	$0/1$	$0/3$	$1/2$	$2/6$	$3/12$	25.0
Visceral	$0/3$	$1/7$	$2/5$	$4/12$	$7/27$	26.0
Total	$0/5$	$1/12$	$4/9$	$11/29$	$16/55$	29.1

further noted that the remission rate from oestrogen therapy for patients more than five years postmenopausal was significantly better than for patients less than five years postmenopausal.

KENNEDY and BROWN (1965) reported the results of a further investigation where stilboestrol and testosterone propionate were given simultaneously to twenty-two patients with advanced breast cancer. Nine of these (40.9 per cent) obtained a remission; a rate comparable to that obtained from stilboestrol alone.

These results indicate the superior effect of stilboestrol over testosterone propionate and have been confirmed by other observers (e. g. Foss, 1956) but all reports have not shown this trend. In the report of the Co-operative Breast Cancer Group (1964 a) it was pointed out that in one of KENNEDY's studies, comparing testosterone propionate with stilboestrol, the response rates from the two drugs were almost identical (4/37 remissions for testosterone propionate compared with 6/33 remissions for stilboestrol). Because of this, a warning was given against attempting to read too much into results obtained from small samples. In fact eight studies, comparing androgens and oestrogens, were reported by the Co-operative Breast Cancer Group (1964 a), including KENNEDY's series mentioned above. In these eight studies, twenty-two out of 221 patients (10 per cent) responded to androgen therapy and thirty-four out of 218 patients (16 per cent) responded to oestrogen therapy; although oestrogens had the advantage, the remission rate following both drugs was extraordinarily low.

The American Medical Association report (1960) summarised the comparative response to androgen and oestrogen therapy thus:

"The dilemma may be epitomised by stating that a biological system conditioned for a dominant response to feminisation will tolerate more kindly the insults of its untimely resurgence than it will the physiological travesty of a reversal in sexual polarity." (Sic).

5. The Place of Androgens in Prophylaxis

Castration carried out at the time of mastectomy may postpone the onset of recurrence (see pp. 15—19). In the advanced disease therapeutic castration or androgen therapy seem equally effective and result in about the same remission rate; they are probably alternatives, and work to the same degree in the same type of patient. Possibly androgen therapy and castration are also alternatives as prophylactic measures in the early disease.

The first report of androgen therapy used clinically for this purpose was recorded by PRUDENTE (1945). He administered fairly high doses of testosterone propionate (up to 175 mg per week) to women who had had a radical mastectomy for early breast cancer. PRUDENTE selected his patients by the histological grade of malignancy of the tumour and reported very successful results. He claimed that there was . . . "100 per cent better survival at three, four and five years after the operation." Whilst admitting that there were considerable side effects and that fifty per cent of his women showed signs of virilisation, including disturbances of menstruation— often progressing to amenorrhea—he concluded that the side effects were of secondary importance when the degree of benefit was taken into account.

PRUDENTE's trial was not controlled, his cases were highly selected and his results were compared with those from series that were certainly not comparable. But this does not mean that his claims were unjustified. Androgens may well be of value in the early case—and, if virilisation could be reduced to the minimum, androgens might be a preferable form of prophylaxis to castration.

Further evidence that androgen therapy might be of value after mastectomy was supplied by BULBROOK and his colleagues. They had previously shown that the urinary excretion of aetiocholanolone and 17-OHCS in women with advanced breast cancer could be correlated with the subsequent response to adrenalectomy or hypophysectomy. When the levels of these substances were expressed in a formula known as a discriminant function, a positive number (a positive discriminant) resulted when the urinary levels of aetiocholanolone were high and the 17-OHCS were low; a negative number (a negative discriminant) resulted from low levels of aetiocholanolone and high levels of 17-OHCS. Patients with positive discriminants were likely to benefit from ablation and patients with negative discriminants were likely to fail to respond (see pp. 57—66). The levels of aetiocholanolone were found to be low also in some patients with the early disease (BULBROOK et al., 1962) and calculation of the discriminant function revealed it to be negative in these cases. When the distribution of the discriminant function according to age in patients with early breast cancer was compared with the distribution in patients with advanced breast cancer, the scatter was found to be very similar (Figs. 8 and 9). It had been shown that patients with advanced breast cancer with negative discriminants responded badly to endocrine ablation (BULBROOK et al., 1960) and so a study was planned to investigate the fate of patients with a negative discriminant at mastectomy.

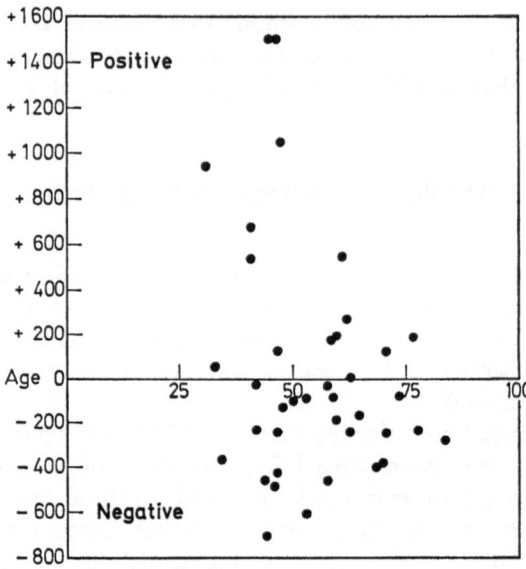

Fig. 8. The discriminant function in patients with early breast cancer

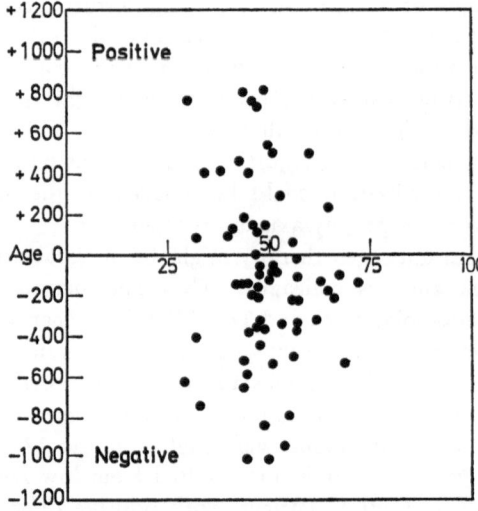

Fig. 9. The discriminant function in patients with advanced breast cancer

In 1964, BULBROOK, HAYWARD and THOMAS were able to report on the follow-up of forty-seven women whose discriminant function had been determined at the time of mastectomy. Each of these patients had had a radical mastectomy for a stage 1 or stage 2 carcinoma of the breast and their hormone assays had been carried out on urine collected on the tenth post-operative day. Twenty-six of the patients were found to have a negative discriminant and twenty-one a positive discriminant. Over 50 per cent of the patients who were discriminant negative at mastectomy had recurred at three years, compared with only 20 per cent of those who were discriminant

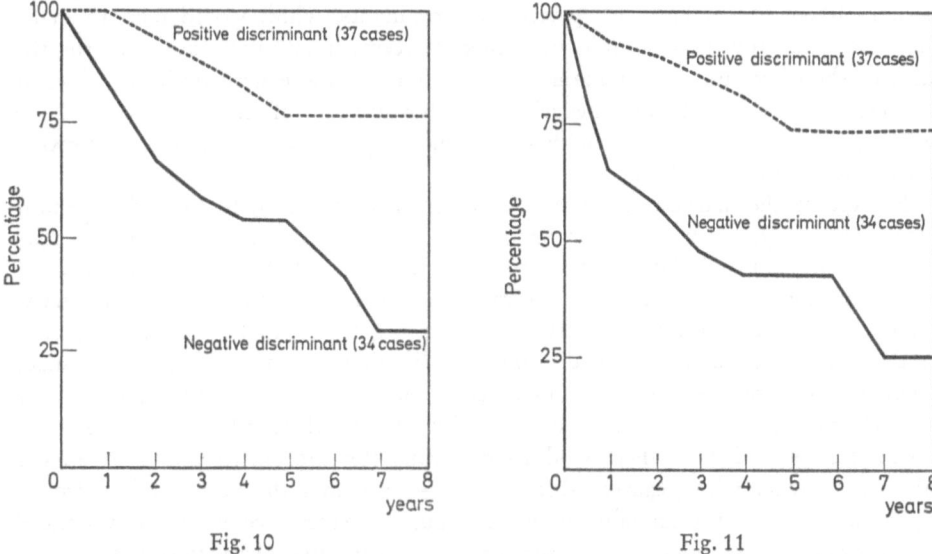

Fig. 10. Proportions free from recurrence up to 8 years after mastectomy in patients with positive and negative discriminants

Fig. 11. Proportions surviving up to 8 years after mastectomy in patients with positive and negative discriminants

positive. Similarly, 45 per cent of the discriminant negative patients had died within three years, compared with less than 10 per cent of those who were discriminant positive. These results were not due to differences in the grade or stage of the tumour and patients with a positive discriminant had tumours of a similar stage and grade to those with negative discriminants. A further report (HAYWARD and BULBROOK, 1968) described the recurrence and survival experience of seventy-one patients up to eight years after mastectomy. Figs. 10 and 11 were calculated by the life table technique and show that the patients with negative discriminants had three times the recurrence and mortality rate at eight years, compared with those with positive discriminants.

It seems that patients with low aetiocholanolone and high 17-OHCS values—and hence negative discriminants—may have both a poor prognosis after mastectomy and a poor subsequent response to endocrine ablation. Conversely, those with positive discriminants at mastectomy tend to have a good prognosis and recur late; if their recurrent disease is subsequently treated with adrenalectomy or hypophysectomy they respond well. This is always presuming that the discriminant remains constant throughout the disease—which it almost certainly does not. BULBROOK and HAYWARD (1965) have described some preliminary results on the value of the discriminant, measured at various times and on various patients between mastectomy and ablation. The mean value of the discriminant remained fairly constant for three years after mastectomy. During this period, those patients whose disease had recurred and who had subsequently died (and, therefore, no longer had their discriminants measured) would be more likely to be those with negative discriminants (see paragraph above). Thus as time progressed after mastectomy, the remaining patient population would be more likely to be that with positive discriminants, which would tend to make the mean value for the discriminant higher. It seems likely, therefore, that for the value of the discriminant to remain constant, some of those with positive values at mastectomy must have become negative in a shorter space of time than would have been expected from experience with the normal population (BULBROOK, HAYWARD, SPICER and THOMAS, 1962 b).

Because of the marked correlation between urinary steroid levels and prognosis after mastectomy, an investigation has been started to test the use of additive hormone therapy as prophylaxis (BULBROOK and HAYWARD, 1965). Treated and control groups are being studied, both of which have the discriminant measured at mastectomy and at regular intervals afterwards. Information should be obtained, both on the predictive value of the discriminant (in those randomised to the control group) and on whether the discriminant could be of value in selecting patients for prophylactic therapy (in those randomised for additive therapy). In the latter case, it is interesting to debate whether additive therapy (by androgens) would have more value in patients with negative discriminants—in whom the additional androgen might convert the discriminant to positive but by experience with the advanced disease would be expected to have hormonally unresponsive tumours—or in patients with positive discriminants—who are presumed to have hormonally responsive tumours and who have a low recurrence rate.

MEAKIN and his colleagues (1968) have described this trial in further detail. All patients aged under fifty, having a mastectomy for a stage 1 or 2 carcinoma of the breast, are being included. Ten days after operation, they are being randomly selected for either a treatment or a control group. Those that are allocated to the control group have no prophylactic therapy, whereas those that enter the treatment group have a 200 mg testosterone implant inserted on the twelfth post-operative day. Further implants are then inserted at nine monthly intervals. It is estimated that this regime will provide the patients with approximately 1 mg of testosterone a day. A careful watch is being kept for signs of virilisation and a record is being made of the patients' menstrual history. The urine samples are being collected both from the treatment and from the control groups two days before mastectomy, ten days after mastectomy and then at six monthly intervals. These samples will be used to estimate the discriminant function. Information should be obtained not only on the value of prophylactic androgen therapy in patients with positive and negative discriminants, but also on the changes in the value of the discriminant after mastectomy. No results are yet available from this trial.

6. Mode of Action

The empiricism with which hormones are used to treat advanced breast cancer continues. Over seventy years have elapsed since alteration in the hormonal environment was found to affect the growth rate of advanced breast cancer and even now there seems to be little evidence on the mechanisms involved. There is probably more ignorance on the mode of action of administered hormones than on the changes that follow ablative procedures. If the ovaries are removed, a fairly reasonable hypothesis would be that the cancer is affected, either directly or indirectly, as a result of the deprivation of the hormones synthesised in the ovaries. Similar presumptions can be made following removal of the pituitary and adrenal glands. Androgen or oestrogen therapy involves the oral or intramuscular administration of synthetic hormones. It is not known whether these synthetic hormones act centrally, by affecting the natural secretion of hormones by the pituitary, adrenals and ovaries, or peripherally by action on the breast and breast tumour.

Some information on the interaction of hormone and target tissue, can be got from measuring the tissue uptake of administered hormones. Steroids which have been labelled, either with 14 carbon or tritium, can be given to patients or animals and subsequently the tissues to be studied can be biopsied. Measurement of the radioactivity of the biopsy specimens gives an indication of the amount of labelled steroid which has been taken up by each tissue. Comparison of the radioactivity of different tissues (e. g. tumour, normal breast, fat, skin and muscle) can be made in the same subject. This will give information on differential uptake. Also, in different subjects, the interval between giving the hormone and taking the biopsy can be varied. If this time is short, the immediate uptake of the tissues can be measured; if the time is long, an estimate can be obtained of how long different tissues retain the administered steroid.

Much of the early work on the action of hormones on target organs was done in animals. JENSEN and JACOBSON (1962) gave oestradiol-17β to rats and noted that the uterus could retain the steroid for as long as six hours after injection. KING et al. (1965) reported that animal tumours induced by dimethylbenzanthracene also had the ability to retain hormones. This ability to retain hormones against a concentration gradient is a property of some target organs. This type of experiment is difficult to carry out in man because of the ethical problem of obtaining tissue biopsies after hormone administration. In studying breast cancer, this difficulty has been overcome principally by investigating patients who were about to have a mastectomy. The hormone is given before operation and the radical mastectomy specimen provides samples of tumour, normal breast tissue, muscle, fat and skin. Admittedly the breast tissue obtained from such a specimen can only be presumed to be normal, an assumption which may be far from the truth.

Using this system, ELLIS et al. (1965) administered tritiated testosterone to thirty-four women before mastectomy. They then measured the radioactivity in tumour, breast, muscle and fat. When the results were expressed in terms of activity per unit wet weight, the uptake of the testosterone by the tumour was more than that of the normal breast—although not significantly so. The uptake of tumour and breast was significantly higher than fat or muscle. On first consideration, the former finding seemed unreasonable. Why should a tissue which has become de-differentiated and lost most of the more sophisticated properties of its parent tissue behave in a more specialised manner in its uptake of hormones? The answer may well be in the use of wet weight as a unit of measurement. Almost certainly—although not as yet proved—epithelial tissue takes up more hormone than connective tissue. Per unit weight, there are usually far more epithelial cells in tumour tissue than in the normal resting breast. These tumour cells may be more primitive and have a diminished affinity for hormones but would be present in sufficient numbers to account for the greater overall uptake by the tumour compared with the normal breast. Suggestive confirmatory evidence of the role of the epithelial cells in hormone uptake is provided by the extremely low counts that are obtained from fat and muscle—tissues composed solely of connective tissue.

ELLIS et al. (1965) investigated the cell uptake of their specimens by carrying out cell counts on sections taken from tumour and normal breast tissue. For tumours, the mean cell count per unit area was 216 compared with 28 for breast tissue—a difference of over sevenfold. By dividing the counts, per minute per gram weight, by the cell count per unit area, a measure of the cell uptake was calculated. When the results were expressed in terms of cell uptake rather than as uptake per unit wet weight, the radioactivity in normal breast was significantly higher than in tumour tissue—the converse of what was found using wet weight, and a result that would seem meaningful. They further noted that in anaplastic tumours, the cell uptake was low. Of the four Grade III tumours in their series (and hence those with least differentiation and the greatest numbers of mitoses), three had a very low uptake of testosterone.

Other workers have not been able to demonstrate the same differences in androgen uptake between tumour and normal breast. BRAUNSBERG, IRVING and JAMES (1967) administered tritiated testosterone to patients who were about to have a mastectomy for breast cancer. In an attempt to achieve tissue equilibrium with the endogenous hormones, they administered the testosterone by constant infusion. The concentrations in the tissues were measured by unit wet weight. They were unable to demonstrate differential uptake by tumour tissue compared with muscle, fat, normal breast or skin, and furthermore, they were unable to find a significant correlation between the tritium concentrations and the cellular and fibrous content of the tumour as estimated by microscopy.

QUINCY and GRAY (1966) also measured the uptake of androgens in the breast. Six hours before operation, they gave tritiated 17 C-methyltestosterone orally to nine patients and measured the radioactivity in tumour, muscle, skin and fat removed from the mastectomy specimen. They observed no difference in the concentration of methyl testosterone in tumour and the other tissues but detected a significantly higher concentration of the metabolites of methyl testosterone in tumour compared with muscle and probably also compared with skin and fat.

DESHPANDE et al. (1966 a) investigated how the mode of administration of labelled testosterone affected tissue uptake. They considered that a single dose of testosterone was unphysiological and that a more normal presentation to the target organs would be obtained by a continuous infusion of the steroid. They gave an infusion of tritium labelled testosterone and a single dose of C^{14} labelled testosterone to the same patients. Measurement of the radioactivity of breast, tumour and fat showed that the uptake was identical following either method of administration. Similar results were reported by DESHPANDE et al. (1966 b) using progesterone. They compared the uptake of labelled progesterone administered by infusion with the uptake when the progesterone was given in a single dose. Again they could detect little difference in the pattern in tumour, normal breast, fat and muscle. They further correlated the uptake of labelled progesterone with the time interval between the administration of the drug and subsequent biopsy. They concluded from their results that breast tissue was able to retain progesterone for a much longer time than neoplastic tissue.

Comparatively more work has been done using labelled oestrogens, and here many reports have indicated preferential uptake by tumour tissue. CROWLEY et al. (1962) gave oestradiol-4-14 C to patients with breast cancer; they found that the radioactivity per unit wet weight was greater in the tumour than in the normal breast. They also noted that tumour with a high connective tissue content picked

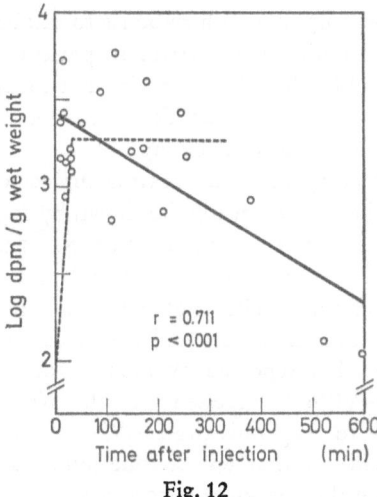
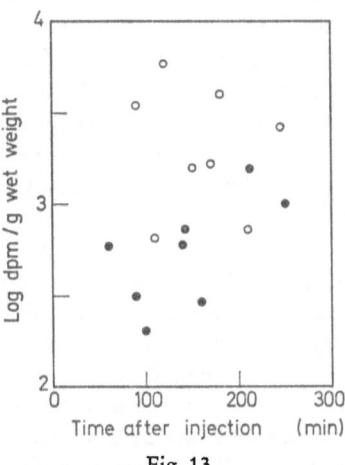

Fig. 12   Fig. 13

Fig. 12. The uptake of radioactivity by tumour tissue after administration of 3H—oestra-diol—17β. The solid line represents the calculated regression of log uptake on time, and the broken line the probable physiological pattern of uptake. (DESHPANDE et al., 1967; reproduced with permission)

Fig. 13. The effect of pretreatment with drostanolone propionate on the uptake of 3H—oestradiol—17β by tumour tissue. (DESHPANDE et al., 1967; reproduced with permission)

up correspondingly little labelled steroid—an observation that again suggests the prime role of the epithelial cell. BRAUNSBERG et al. (1967) administered oestradiol-4-14 C by constant infusion to patients before mastectomy. They noted that a high proportion of the tumours appeared to concentrate oestradiol or its metabolites, whereas this was not observed in normal breast, muscle or skin. DE HERTOGH and PEARLMAN (1964) measured the unit weight radioactivity after an infusion of radioactive oestrone. Conversely, they were unable to detect any significant difference in the uptake of tumour compared with fat and normal breast.

DESHPANDE et al. (1967) gave labelled oestradiol 17β to patients before mastectomy. They again showed that when measured by unit wet weight the tumour contained more radioactivity than normal breast tissue. Of more interest, however, was their observation that there might be a plateau of uptake for both tumour and normal breast tissue. This seemed to last from ten minutes to five hours after administration of the steroid and was followed by a rapid loss of radioactivity (Fig. 12). They likened this pattern of uptake and subsequent discharge of oestradiol 17β by the breast and tumour to that noted by JENSEN and JACOBSON (1962) for the rat uterus.

In a further eight patients, DESHPANDE et al. (1967) gave a single dose of drostanolone propionate (an androgen of known effect in treating the advanced disease) eighteen hours before mastectomy. Within five hours of mastectomy, these patients were also given tritiated oestradiol 17β. The uptake of the oestradiol was then measured in tumour and breast tissue and compared with the uptake of patients not pre-treated with drostanolone. This comparison produced rather startling results. The drostanolone had no apparent effect on the accumulation of oestradiol 17β by the normal breast, but there was about a 75 per cent reduction in the uptake by the tumour (Fig. 13). The implications of this finding are as yet unknown.

One attempt has been made to associate tissue uptake with response to subsequent treatment. FOLCA, GLASCOCK and IRVINE gave tritiated hexoestrol to patients with advanced metastatic breast cancer. They then biopsied skin deposits and measured the radioactivity. Some correlation was noted between the uptake of the secondary deposits and the response of the patient to subsequent adrenalectomy.

In vitro studies have not proved so satisfactory in demonstrating differences in steroid uptake by different tissues. Or rather, the pattern of uptake shown by *in vitro* studies has not correlated with that found using *in vivo* studies. BRAUNSBERG and JAMES (1967) investigated the uptake of labelled testosterone, oestradiol and progesterone by normal tissue and breast cancer *in vitro*. They noted that the adipose tissue took up more testosterone than muscle, normal breast and breast carcinoma, a finding which was the complete opposite of that reported by ELLIS et al. (1965) using *in vivo* studies. BRAUNSBERG and JAMES (1967) suggested that the affinity of steroid for adipose tissue *in vitro* may be due to the lipids present. They were also unable to demonstrate in their system any evidence that testosterone influenced the uptake of oestradiol or that oestradiol influenced the uptake of testosterone.

So far, these investigations have thrown little light on the problem of how administered hormones act when used to treat advanced breast cancer. Few of the labelled steroids that have been administered are used in treatment and much of the work done on them can be interpreted in many different ways. It seems that little further will come out of this approach until certain fundamental questions have been answered. Of particular importance is an answer to the problem of how the uptake of tissues should be expressed; should the measurements be given in terms of wet weight, in terms of cell uptake or in terms of some other index—for example DNA content? Expressions of activity using unit wet weight and cell uptake give diametrically opposite results and it would seem that further studies to determine the actual site of uptake within the tissues and within the cell must be made before the results will be meaningful.

But some progress has been made. It has been shown that both breast and breast tumour can act as target organs in the uptake of oestradiol 17β although not apparently in the uptake of progesterone and certain androgens. Furthermore the uptake of oestradiol by tumour tissue may be influenced by the previous administration of androgens. Perhaps most important of all, attention has now been directed back to the tumour and its parent tissue. The availability of assays for the measurement of blood and urinary steroids have for long encouraged research workers to investigate the hormonal environment. Measurements of the hormonal environment are certainly important but the results may be meaningless without a parallel knowledge of the behaviour of the tissue on which this environment acts.

7. Hypercalcaemia

Patients with breast cancer who are on hormone therapy sometimes have raised levels of serum calcium. In one of the very early papers on the therapeutic use of hormones, FARROW and WOODARD (1942) found the problems of hypercalcaemia so difficult that they condemned androgens as a treatment for the advanced disease.

The first observations on hypercalcaemia in malignant disease were probably made by VIRCHOW in 1855 and it has now been recognised as a common complication of many cancers. MEAKIN (1967) lists breast, bronchus, lymphosarcoma, multiple myeloma, cervix and kidney as being the six most commonly associated neoplasms. He found hypercalcaemia to be most common in patients with breast cancer but this was mainly because breast cancer is a common tumour. Relatively speaking, patients with multiple myeloma are more at risk.

There are two principal types of hypercalcaemia associated with neoplasia:

1. When there are widespread skeletal deposits and the hypercalcaemia is a simple expression of bone destruction, calcium is liberated into the blood stream at a faster rate than it can be excreted through the kidney.

2. When the hypercalcaemia is unrelated to skeletal metastases. In this type, there may also be a concomitant depression of serum phosphorus.

It is the latter type of hypercalcaemia that is most interesting scientifically. It seems to occur in two forms, dependent on the levels of serum phosphorus.

a) Hypercalcaemia in Patients without Skeletal Metastases and with Depressed Levels of Serum Phosphorus

This is commonly associated with carcinoma of the bronchus or kidney but it is not encountered in patients with breast tumours. It has been suggested that the condition may be due to an excess of parathormone, but there is little evidence to support this and it seems more likely that the tumour itself is secreting a parathormone-like substance. Evidence for this includes the low serum phosphorus, diminished tubular reabsorption of phosphate and the fact that the serum calcium is depressed following successful anti-tumour treatment, only to rise again when that treatment is stopped. The lowered serum phosphorus will be seen only in the presence of normal renal function. If the hypercalcaemia has caused renal failure, the phosphorus levels may be normal. Experimental work seems to confirm that the tumour is producing a hormone. MEAKIN (1967) records that MUNSON, TASHJIAN and LEVINE (1965) and SHERWOOD (1966) have identified a parathormone-like molecule from tumour tissue taken from hypercalcaemia patients. In the blood of one such patient, hyperparathyroid ranges of parathormone were detected.

b) Hypercalcaemia in Patients without Skeletal Metastases and with Normal Serum Phosphorus

This may occur in patients who are hypercalcaemic as in (a) above, when there is associated renal damage. The renal damage interfers with the excretion of phosphorus, resulting in normal levels of phosphorus being found in the serum. In patients with breast cancer, hypercalcaemia with normal serum phosphorus may occur without evidence of renal damage; under these circumstances, there is evidence that the tumour is producing an oesteolytic substance but different from the parathormone-like substance described above. Experimentally, when the tumour is implanted subcutaneously over the skull of a rat, local bony reabsorption will occur. Furthermore a lipid extract of this tumour can be prepared which when administered to the parathyroidectomised rat can induce osteolysis and hypercalcuria (GORDAN et al., 1966). Chemically, it is similar but not identical to 7-dehydrotachysterol which is a precursor of vitamin D3. Two osteolytic sterols have been extracted from human breast cancer tissue and from plasma; these have now been positively identified as Δ^7 sitosteryl acetate and sigmesteryl acetate (GORDAN, 1967).

To summarise, therefore, there are three distinct causes of hypercalcaemia in patients with cancer:

1. Associated with widespread skeletal metastases when the hypercalcaemia is a reflection of the rate of mobilisation of calcium from bone and the rate of excretion by the kidney.

2. Without skeletal metastases but with a decreased serum phosphorus (if renal function is normal) which is probably due to a parathormone-like substance produced by the tumour.

3. Without skeletal metastases and with a normal serum phosphorus, probably due to a liberation of a Vitamin D3 like substance from the tumour.

Clinically hypercalcaemia either occurs spontaneously or it can be associated with the beginning of hormone therapy. Its presentation is protean and MEAKIN (1967) has listed the symptoms and signs as:

A. Nervous System
   1. Personality changes, lethargy, etc.
   2. Anorexia, nausea and vomiting
   3. Paraesthesiae
   4. Depressed tendon reflexes

B. Skeletal Muscle
   1. Weakness
   2. Hypotonia
   3. Depressed tendon reflexes

C. Smooth Muscle
   1. Anorexia
   2. Constipation

D. Kidney
   1. Polyuria   (a) Osmotic
                  (b) Interference with concentration
                  (c) Chronic renal failure
   2. Polydipsia
   3. Renal failure
   4. Nephrolithiasis

E. Heart
   Shortened Q. T. interval

F. Metastatic calcification (kidney, cornea, stomach, lung, etc.)

When hypercalcaemia occurs spontaneously, treatment must be aimed at the tumour itself. Whether the hypercalcaemia is caused by the tumour invading bone or by the tumour producing a specific hormone, successful treatment will result in the serum calcium levels falling. Empirically it has been found that high doses of steroids (Prednisone 25—50 mg daily) are most satisfactory in the rapid depression of serum calcium levels. It is not known whether these steroids act directly on the growth or indirectly involving other endocrine changes.

It is also important to correct the dehydration that accompanies hypercalcaemia and this can be satisfactorily accomplished by the intravenous infusion of a solution of sodium chloride. More effective than this, however, may be the use of a solution of sodium sulphate. WALSER and BROWDER (1959) originally noted in the dog that urinary calcium excretion was greatly increased by an infusion of sodium sulphate. This hypercalcuria occurred to such an extent as to induce hypocalcaemia in the normal animal. Sodium sulphate appeared to be five times more effective than sodium chloride in clearing the blood of calcium.

Subsequently, CHAKNAKJLAN and BETHUNE (1966) demonstrated the value of sodium sulphate clinically in the treatment of hypercalcaemia.

Neither treatment with prednisone nor the infusion with sodium sulphate are necessarily effective in every case and it is not yet known what are the specific indications for each therapy. DONOVAN et al. (1966) described one patient in whom therapy with prednisone was successful when sodium sulphate had failed and another patient in whom the exact converse occurred.

Inorganic phosphate has also been given successfully to treat hypercalcaemia secondary to malignant disease. The phosphate can be given by mouth or, if vomiting is a problem, intravenously. Some series report a lowering of the serum calcium in all patients receiving treatment, without an associated rise in the serum phosphate (THALASSINOS and JOPLIN, 1968). The treatment has no serious side effects and, as was once feared, extraskeletal calcification is not a problem.

When hypercalcaemia results from the administration of hormones, it is important that the drugs be stopped immediately. This may be sufficient to bring the calcium levels back to normal and then an alternative treatment may be applied. On the other hand, it may be necessary to apply specific treatment to combat the hypercalcaemia—such as prednisone, sodium sulphate or phosphate—as described above. DONOVAN et al. (1966) suggested that when androgens or oestrogens are being considered as therapy in the presence of osseous metastases, the initial dose should be small and gradually increased. The treatment should be stopped if any abnormality develops in the serum calcium, and an alternative therapy tried.

Summary and Conclusions

1. Hormones give effective palliation in more than 20 per cent of patients with advanced breast cancer; in successful cases the survival is slightly increased.

2. The histological changes in responding lesions are similar to those following radiation therapy, but viable malignant cells survive even when the tumour is in complete regression.

3. The response to hormone therapy is probably a property of the tumour. So far, new compounds have not given a higher response rate than testosterone or stilboestrol although the side effects may be less.

4. Androgens should be used in women who are premenopausal or are up to 5 years postmenopausal. Oestrogens should be used in women more than 5 years postmenopausal. The response to oestrogens and probably to androgens increases with advancing age.

5. The dose of androgens or oestrogens which will give an optimum response is not known, but very small doses of oestrogens probably stimulate the tumour.

6. Patients with visceral metastases have the lowest incidence of remission but this may be due to debility. The site of the metastases should not influence the choice of hormone.

7. Rapidly growing tumours (indicated by a short free period and large size of primary) have a low response rate, but there is no reliable correlation between response and other macroscopic or microscopic features of the tumour.

8. There is no direct evidence on the mode of action of androgens or oestrogens in inhibiting breast cancer. Both the breast and breast tumour can act as target organs and take up circulating hormones differentially.

9. Hypercalcaemia is a particular hazard to patients with breast cancer treated with hormones. It is caused, either by widespread osteolytic deposits, or by a specific osteolytic sterol produced by the breast tumour. It can be treated by high doses of steroid, by hydration and by the administration of phosphates.

References

BRAUNSBERG, H., IRVINE, W. T., JAMES, V. H. T.: A comparison of steroid hormone concentrations in human tissues including breast cancer. Brit. J. Cancer 21, 714 (1967).

— JAMES, V. H. T.: Observations on the binding of testosterone to malignant mammary tumours and other tissues in vitro. Brit. J. Cancer 21, 703 (1967).

BULBROOK, R. D., GREENWOOD, F. C., HAYWARD, J. L.: Selection of breast cancer patients for adrenalectomy or hypophysectomy by determination of urinary 17-hydroxy corticosteroids and aetiocholanolone. Lancet 1960 I, 1154.

— HAYWARD, J. L.: The possibility of predicting the response of patients with early breast cancer to subsequent endocrine ablation. Cancer Res. 25, 1135 (1965).

— — SPICER, C. C., THOMAS, B. S.: Abnormal excretion of urinary steroids by women with early breast cancer. Lancet 1962 a II, 1238.

— — — — A comparison between the urinary steroid excretion of normal women and women with advanced breast cancer. Lancet 1962 b II, 1235.

— — THOMAS, B. S.: The relation between the urinary 17-hydroxy corticosteroids and 11-deoxy-17-oxosteroids and the fate of patients after mastectomy. Lancet 1964 I, 945.

CANTINO, I. J., GORDAN, G. S.: High dosage Δ_1 testolactone therapy of disseminated carcinoma of the breast. Cancer 20, 458 (1967).

CHAKMAKJIAN, Z. H., BETHUNE, J. E.: Sodium sulfate treatment of hypercalcemia. New Engl. J. Med. 275, 862 (1966).

Co-operative Breast Cancer Group: Results of studies of the Co-operative Breast Cancer Group 1961—1963. Cancer Chemother. Rep. 41, Suppl. 1 (1964 a).

Co-operative Breast Cancer Group: Testosterone Propionate Therapy in Breast Cancer. J. Amer. med. Ass. 188, 1069 (1964 b).

Council on Drugs, Subcommittee on Breast and Genital Cancer, Committee on Research, American Medical Association: Androgens and Oestrogens in the treatment of disseminated mammary carcinoma; retrospective study of 944 patients. J. Amer. med. Ass. 172, 1271 (1960).

Council on Pharmacy and Chemistry. Current status of hormone therapy of advanced mammary cancer. J. Amer. med. Ass. 146, 471 (1951).

CROWLEY, L. G., DEMETRIOU, J., MacDONALD, I., KOTIN, P., KUSHINSKY, S., DONOVAN, A. J.: Levels of exogenous oestrogens in tissues in human mammary carcinoma. Surg. Forum 13, 103 (1962).

CUTLER, M., SCHLEMENSON, M.: Treatment of advanced mammary cancer with testosterone. J. Amer. med. Ass. 138, 187 (1948).

CUTLER, S. J.: In: Clinical Evaluation in Breast Cancer. Eds.: J. L. HAYWARD and R. D. BULBROOK. London-New York: Academic Press 1966, p. 214.

DE HERTOGH, R., PEARLMAN, W. H.: Metabolism and Localisation of Estrone-6,7-H³ in Breast Cancer. Fed. Proc. 23, 276 (1964).

DESHPANDE, N., BULBROOK, R. D., BELZER, F. O.: Comparison between uptake of radioactivity by normal and neoplastic human breast tissue after single injection and intravenous infusion of tritiated testosterone. J. Endocr. 34, 125 (1966 a).

— — — An apparent selective accumulation of progesterone by the human breast. Excerpta Medica Internat. Congress. Series No. 132, 750 (1966 b).

— JENSEN, V., BULBROOK, R. D.: Accumulation of triated oestradiol by human breast tissue. Steroids 10, 219 (1967).

Donovan, A. J., Bethune, J. E., Berne, T. V.: Hypercalcaemia in patients with advanced mammary cancer and osseous metastases. Effect of hormone therapy and schedule of treatment. Amer. Surg. 32, 673 (1966).

Douglas, M.: The treatment of advanced breast cancer by hormone therapy. Brit. J. Cancer 6, 32 (1952).

Ellis, F., Parker, J. R., Bulbrook, R. D., Deshpande, N.: The uptake of radioactivity by normal and neoplastic human breast tissues after administration of tritiated testosterone. Brit. J. Surg. 52, 54 (1965).

Emerson, W. J., Kennedy, B. J., Graham, J. N., Nathanson, I. T.: Pathology of primary and recurrent carcinoma of the human breast after administration of steroid hormones. Cancer 6, 641 (1953).

Farrow, J. H., Woodard, H. Q.: The influence of Androgenic and Estrogenic substances on serum calcium. J. Amer. med. Ass. 118, 339 (1942).

Folca, P. J., Glascock, R. F., Irvine, W. T.: Studies with tritium labelled hexoestrol in advanced breast cancer. Lancet 1961 II, 796.

Foss, G. L.: Palliative hormone therapy of advanced mammary cancer. Lancet 1956 I, 651.

Galton, D. A. G.: Androgen therapy in 70 cases of advanced mammary carcinoma. Brit. J. Cancer 4, 20 (1950).

Goldenberg, I. S.: Testosterone propionate therapy in breast cancer. J. Amer. med. Ass. 188, 1069 (1964).

— Bailar, J. C., Lowry, R.: Survival of women with hormonally treated breast cancer. Surg. Gynec. Obstet. 119, 785 (1964).

Gordan, G. S.: Hormonal effects of nonendocrine tumors with special reference to the hypercalcemia of breast cancer. In: Current Concepts in Breast Cancer. Eds.: A. Segaloff, K. K. Meyers, and S. DeBakey. Baltimore: Williams & Wilkins 1967, p. 132.

— Cantino, R. J., Erhardt, L., Hansen, J., Lubich, W.: Osteolytic sterol in human breast cancer. Science 151, 1226 (1966).

Gowing, N. F. C.: Histological changes in response to therapy. In: Clinical Evaluation in Breast Cancer. Eds.: J. L. Hayward and R. D. Bulbrook. London-New York: Academic Press 1966, p. 53.

Hayward, J. L.: An evaluation of some factors affecting oestrogen response in the treatment of advanced cancer of the breast. Guy's Hosp. Rep. 106, 254 (1957).

— Assessment of response to treatment at Guy's Hospital Breast Clinic. The estimation of the Mean Clinical Value. In: Clinical Evaluation in Breast Cancer. Eds.: J. L. Hayward and R. D. Bulbrook. London-New York: Academic Press 1966, pp. 131, 285.

— Bulbrook, R. D.: Urinary steroids and prognosis in breast cancer. In: Prognostic Factors in Breast Cancer. Eds.: A. P. M. Forrest and P. B. Kunkler. Edinburgh-London: Livingstone 1968, p. 383.

Jensen, E. V., Jacobson, H. I.: Basic guides to the mechanism of estrogen action. Recent Progr. Hormone Res. 18, 387 (1962).

Kennedy, B. J.: Diethylstilbestrol versus testosterone therapy in advanced breast cancer. Surg. Gynec. Obstet. 120, 1246 (1965).

— Hormone therapy for advanced breast cancer. Cancer 18, 1551 (1965).

— Brown, J. H.: Combined estrogenic and androgenic hormone therapy in advanced breast cancer. Cancer 18, 431 (1965).

King, R. J., Cowan, D. M., Inman, D. R.: The uptake of (6.7-3-H) oestradiol by dimethylbenzathracene-induced rat mammary tumours.

Koller, P. C.: Influences of synthetic oestrogens upon advanced malignant disease. Addendum to A. Haddow, J. M. Watkinson, and E. Paterson. Brit. med. J. 1944 II, 393.

Lewison, E. L., Trimble, F. H.: Advanced mammary carcinoma, treated with sex hormones. J. Amer. med. Ass. 162, 1429 (1956).

Meakin, J. W.: Personal Communication (1967).

— Allt, W. E. C., Beale, F. A., Brown, T. C., Bulbrook, R. D., Clark, R. M., Fitzpatrick, P. J., Hawkins N. V., Hayward, J. L., Jenkins, R. D. T.: A preliminary report of two studies of adjuvant treatment of primary breast cancer. In: Prognostic Factors in Breast Cancer. Eds.: A. P. M. Forrest and P. B. Kunkler. Edinburgh-London: Livingstone 1968, p. 157.

MUNSON, P. L., TASHJIAN, A. H., LEVINE, L.: Evidence for parathyroid hormone in non-parathyroid tumours associated with hypercalcemia. Cancer Res. **25**, 1062 (1965).

NATHANSON, I. T.: Hormones in relation to tumours of the female. Prog. Gynaecology **2**, 218 (1950).

PRUDENTE, A.: Postoperative prophyllaxis of recurrent mammary cancer with testosterone propionate. Surg. Gynec. Obstet. **80**, 575 (1945).

QUINCEY, R. V., GRAY, C. H.: Uptake of (1,2-^{3}H) 17α Methyltestosterone by breast carcinoma and other tissues of human subjects. Brit. J. Cancer 20, 271 (1966).

SEGALOFF, A.: Assessment of response to treatment by the Co-operative Breast Cancer Group. In: Clinical Evaluation in Breast Cancer. Eds.: J. L. HAYWARD and R. D. BULBROOK. London-New York: Academic Press 1966, pp. 125, 275.

— Hormones and breast cancer. Recent Progr. Hormone Res. **22**, 351 (1966).

— HORWITT, B. N., CARABISI, R. A., MURISON, P. J., SCHLOSSER, J. V.: Hormonal therapy in cancer of the breast. V. The effect of methyltestosterone on clinical course and hormonal excretion. Cancer **6**, 483 (1953).

— WEETH, J. B., MEYER, K. K., RONGONE, E. L., CUNNINGHAM, M. E. G.: Hormonal therapy in cancer of the breast. XIX. Effect of oral administration of Δ_1 testololactone on clinical course and hormone excretion. Cancer **15**, 633 (1962).

— — RONGONE, E. L., MURISON, P. J., BOWERS, C. Y.: Hormonal therapy in cancer of the breast. XVI. The effect of Δ_1 testololactone on clinical course and hormonal excretion. Cancer **13**, 1017 (1960).

SHERWOOD, L. M., O'RIORDAN, J. L., AURBACH, G. D.: Production of parathyroid hormone by nonparathyroid tumors. J. clin. Endocr. **27**, 140 (1967).

THALASSINOS, N., JOPLIN, G. F.: Phosphate treatment of hypercalcaemia due to carcinoma. Brit. med. J. **1968** II, 14.

VIRCHOW, R.: Virchows Arch. path. Anat. **8**, 103 (1855).

WALPOLE, A. L., PATERSON, E.: Synthetic oestrogens in mammary cancer. Lancet **1949** II, 783.

WALSER, M., BROWDER, A. A.: Ion association III: The Effect of sulfate infusion on calcium excretion. J. clin. Invest. **38**, 1404 (1959).

WOLFF, B.: The differential cell count in cancer of the breast and response to hormone therapy. Guy's Hosp. Rep. **106**, 53 (1957).

Chapter 6

Corticosteroids and Progestogens

Corticosteroids and progestogens have only recently been used in the treatment of women with advanced breast cancer, and their action is possibly less well understood than that of castration, androgens, oestrogens or the major ablative procedures. There is also less known about the indications for their use and of the degree of remission that can be expected.

1. Corticosteroids

The prescription of corticosteroids is now an accepted treatment for the advanced disease. The compounds have two effects. First, they give an objective remission in a small proportion of cases, and second, they cause a sense of well-being in the patient. Indeed, the subjective response may outweigh the anti-tumour effect. The development of Cushingoid facies and the gain in weight are occasionally disturbing but otherwise there are few side effects.

The use of corticosteroids as treatment probably originates from the doubts of many surgeons about the mechanism of response that followed adrenalectomy or hypophysectomy. Patients having these operations had to be maintained on cortisone replacement therapy and this replacement therapy could have accounted for the remission. Cortisone therapy was tried as treatment for patients with intact adrenal and pituitary glands and found to be effective. The idea grew that by administering cortisone or prednisone a "medical adrenalectomy" was carried out, and that the anti-tumour effect was similar to what could be achieved by the surgical removal of the adrenal glands. Prednisone seemed the drug of choice as there was less conversion *in vivo* to androgenic products (SLAUNWHITE and SANDBERG, 1957). Also the maintenance of a normal salt and water balance was easier with prednisone therapy than with cortisone. The ovaries had to be removed or irradiated because steroid administration did not inhibit ovarian oestrogen secretion. NISSEN-MEYER, one of the originators and a great protagonist of this treatment, reported on forty-three patients treated with cortisone (50 mg a day) and ovarian ablation, either by surgery or irradiation (NISSEN-MEYER and VOGT, 1961). The treatment was considered successful if there was measurable evidence of tumour regression or if the tumour growth was arrested for at least six months. Using these criteria, NISSEN-MEYER and VOGT reported a remission rate of 51 per cent. This remission rate is high and may in part be explained by their interpretation of what constitutes a successful response; in many instances, the tumour regression lasted less than two months. Other series have since been reported and a feature of these has been the wide variation in response rate. For instance, DAO et al. (1961) obtained no response in a series of twenty patients treated with cortisone. SEGALOFF et al. (1954), when treating nineteen patients with either ACTH or cortisone, also noted no success. On the other hand, LEMON (1959) reported a 48 per cent remission rate in thirty one patients, treated with prednisone. But here again, the successful cases included those in whom the progress of the disease was only arrested and also those whose remission lasted less than six months.

The exact effect of administered corticosteroids is not well understood, but their action is probably not confined to the few patients who obtain a response. SHERLOCK and HARTMAN (1962) analysed the pattern of mestastases in 204 patients who were receiving adrenal steroids as additive therapy and compared them with controls. They observed a highly significant increase in the incidence of metastases in the opposite breast, the mucosa of the stomach and duodenum and the spleen and brain. They suggested that this might be due both to a generalised reduction in the host's immune response and to a specific effect of the steroids on certain organs which rendered them more favourable targets for secondary growth. Patients who were receiving corticosteroids as replacement therapy only had an increase in metastases to the spleen.

The beneficial action of corticosteroids on breast cancer is probably the result of their inhibiting effect on the adrenal cortex. NISSEN-MEYER and SVERDRUP (1961) measured the urinary oestrone, oestriol, oestradiol 17β and pregnanediol in breast cancer patients who were either postmenopausal or had been castrated. Fifty-five patients were studied and twenty-five of these were receiving additive steroid therapy. The mean levels of all these hormones were significantly lower in the group receiving steroid therapy, compared with the group not receiving steroids. Oestrogen excretion was not abolished by steroid therapy but this might not indicate that the adrenal glands were still active because oestrogens can still be found in the urine of patients who have had an adrenalectomy and oophorectomy (BULBROOK et al., 1958).

The interesting feature of steroid therapy is not that it produces a remission in some cases of breast cancer but rather that the remission does not approximate more closely to that obtained from surgical removal of the adrenal glands. Controlled series, comparing steroid therapy with adrenalectomy, have been reported by DAO et al. (1961) and by FORREST and his colleagues (1968). In both trials a better remission rate was noted in the patients undergoing adrenalectomy. The reason for this difference in response is not known; possibly the adrenal hormone secretion is not sufficiently depressed by steroid therapy; possibly the secretion of different hormones specifically associated with the growth of breast cancer is not affected to the same degree. JANT et al. (1963) found there was a significantly greater degree of adrenal atrophy after hypophysectomy than after corticosteroid therapy alone. The adreno-cortical atrophy produced by steroid therapy was maximal after fifteen to twenty weeks of continuous administration of a dosage equivalent to 60 mg of cortisone or 15 mg of prednisone per day.

Whatever is the true reason for the difference in remission rates between steroid therapy and ablation, the treatments are not alternatives nor is the response to endocrine ablation simply a measure of the response to the cortisone used as replacement therapy.

Many physicians now reserve treatment by steroids for those patients who are not fit for adrenalectomy or hypophysectomy, either by reason of their age or because of the extent of their disease. Under these circumstances, the subjective improvement, which is so marked in patients receiving steroids, can be used to the best advantage.

2. Progestogens

Interest has only recently turned to the possible use of progestogens as treatment for advanced breast cancer. This has largely resulted from the development and synthesis of orally active compounds, of which the most successful have been the 19-nor-testosterones. Before the introduction of the progestogens, progesterone itself had been tried for the treatment of the advanced disease but even when given orally, in a dose as high as 2 grams per day, it failed to produce a remission (Co-operative Breast Cancer Group, 1964). Over the past few years, numerous new progestogens have been synthesised and are now in clinical use. The motive force in the development of these new compounds has principally been the search for new and improved progestational agents for use with oestrogens in the contraceptive pill. BRIGGS et al. (1967) recently listed twenty three compounds which are now clinically available. Not all progestational compounds are effective in the treatment of human breast cancer and the Co-operative Breast Cancer Group (1964) has reported on several compounds which were shown to have no effect when tested in their screening programme.

The remission rate following progestogen therapy in breast cancer again depends on the criteria used for deciding whether a patient has had a successful response. Many active compounds have been tested by the Co-operative Breast Cancer Group and the results have been analysed by their protocol. In a progress report published in 1961, a 22.3 per cent remission rate was described in 520 cases—a result almost identical to that obtained when using testosterone propionate.

Side effects from the treatment seem few. Thrombophlebitis can occur and occasionally vaginal bleeding has been reported but neither is a serious problem. CROWLEY and MACDONALD (1965) remark that when progestogens are combined with oestrogen therapy, there is a considerable diminution in the amount of oedema that so commonly accompanies the administration of oestrogen alone. Also, rather surprisingly, areolar pigmentation caused by previous oestrogen therapy may decrease or disappear when progestogens are added to the treatment regime. The only side effect of serious consequence is liver damage. STOLL et al. (1966) reported that in four patients receiving Lyndiol (an oral contraceptive containing Lynoestrol and Mestranol), as treatment for advanced breast cancer, there was a rise in the serum glutamic oxalacetic transaminase and isocitric dehydrogenase levels. These changes occured following two weeks of administration of approximately six times the contraceptive dose of Lyndiol and were accompained by jaundice in two of the patients. Liver biopsy on all four patients showed parenchymal cell necrosis in the centrilobular zones. A further seven patients were given the progestogen component of Lyndiol (30 mg Lynoestrol—the equivalent of six tablets) and three of these developed a raised serum transaminase level. Two patients had a liver biopsy which showed similar changes to that observed in the patients taking Lyndiol. Four patients who took only the oestrogen component of the pill showed no abnormalities of the serum transaminase or evidence of liver damage.

Probably, the maximum anti-tumour effect is obtained when progestogens and oestrogens are used together. STOLL (1967) found that contraceptive doses of an oestrogen-progestogen pill gave a remission in four out of twenty one patients. When he administered the progestogen component alone to seven patients, only one had a remission; similarly when he gave the oestrogen alone to four patients, none remitted. None of these series was adequately controlled, nor was the treatment chosen by random sample, so the comparative results should be viewed with some caution.

CROWLEY and MACDONALD (1965) studied twenty two postmenopausal patients who were receiving oestrogen therapy. When the oestrogen therapy failed, Delalutin (a progestogen) was added to the treatment schedule and six out of the twenty two patients had an objective response lasting up to 104 weeks.

The successful use of progestogen therapy, after oestrogen therapy or androgen therapy has failed, has been frequently reported and seems to be a characteristic of the treatment. STOLL (1967) noted a successful response to Lyndiol therapy in patients who had failed to respond to previous androgens or oestrogens. He could detect no correlation between the response to progestational agents and response to previous hormone therapy.

Perhaps the most remarkable reports of the use of progestational agents followed a description by HUGGINS and his colleagues (1962) of the beneficial effect of a combination of oestradiol and progesterone on experimental mammary tumours. LANDAU and his colleagues used the same two drugs on patients with advanced breast cancer and claimed that nine out of fifteen patients benefited from the treatment. Subsequently they changed their treatment to Delalutin (500 mg a week) and oestradiol valerate (40 mg a week) and reported on thirty three patients treated with this combination (LANDAU, 1967). They claimed that nine of the thirty three patients responded to the oestrogen-progestogen treatment and—most significant of all—that many of these patients had previously failed to respond to adrenalectomy or hypophysectomy. This is one of the few times that patients have been shown to react to hormone administration after failing to respond to endocrine ablation. A similar claim has been made by KENNEDY (1965) using a combination of stilboestrol (15 mg a day) and Delalutin (500 mg thrice weekly). He reported an improvement in two out of four patients who had previously relapsed following hypophysectomy.

At the moment, it is difficult to determine the precise place of progestogens in the management of advanced breast cancer. The protagonists of the therapy are enthusiastic about its value in palliation and continue to recommend its use. And yet, for some reason it is not often prescribed in preference to androgens, oestrogens or corticosteroids. It seems from the work of the Co-operative Breast Cancer Group (1961) that progestogens and testosterone propionate give very similar results. With their relative lack of side effects, this should make progestational agents the treatment of choice, at least in pre-menopausal women.

The reports that a response may occur, when a combination of progestogens and oestrogens is used after adrenalectomy or hypophysectomy, are extremely encouraging and mean that something may still be accomplished even at this late stage.

More definitive clinical investigations should be carried out. Much of the work on progestogens has been done on ill-assorted groups of patients so that little meaning can be read into the results. There have been few attempts to compare the response with patients in control groups, receiving more conventional treatment. Until more randomised, controlled, clinical trials are established, there seems to be little hope of progressing further in this subject.

Summary and Conclusions

1. Corticosteroids (with castration in premenopausal patients) produce a remission in a small proportion of patients with advanced breast cancer.

2. The remission is not as good as that obtained from adrenalectomy or hypophysectomy.

3. As additive therapy, corticosteroids should probably be used only on patients who have failed to respond to androgens or oestrogens and who are too ill or too old for ablative procedures.

4. Corticosteroids probably act by inhibiting the adrenal cortex.

5. Progestogens can also cause breast cancer to regress in a small number of cases.

6. Progestogens may give a similar response rate to androgens or oestrogens and with less side effects but this has not yet been proved convincingly by clinical trial.

7. Progestogens may occasionally give a response when adrenalectomy or hypophysectomy have failed.

References

BRIGGS, M. H., CALDWELL, A. D. S., PITCHFORD, A. G.: The treatment of cancer by progestogens. Hospital Medicine 2, 63 (1967).

BULBROOK, R. D., GREENWOOD, F. C., HADFIELD, G. J., SCOWEN, E. F.: Adrenalectomy in breast cancer. An attempt to correlate clinical results with oestrogen production. Brit. med. J. 1958 I, 12.

Co-operative Breast Cancer Group: Results of studies by the Co-operative Breast Cancer Group, 1956—1960. Cancer Chemother. Rep. 11, 109 (1961).

Co-operative Breast Cancer Group: Results of studies of the Co-operative Breast Cancer Group, 1961—1963. Cancer Chemother. Rep. 41, 1 (1964).

CROWLEY, L. G., MACDONALD, I.: Delalutin and Estrogens for the treatment of advanced mammary carcinoma in the postmenopausal women. Cancer 18, 436 (1965).

DAO, T. L., TAN, E., BROOKS, V.: A comparative evaluation of adrenalectomy and cortisone in the treatment of advanced mammary carcinoma. Cancer 14, 1259 (1961).

FORREST, A. P. M., STEWART, H. J., BENSON, E. A., KER, H., JONES, V., KUNKLER, P. B., CAMPBELL, H.: Controlled studies in advanced breast cancer. In: Prognostic Factors in Breast Cancer. Eds.: A. P. M. FORREST and P. B. KUNKLER. Edinburgh-London: Livingstone 1968, p. 186.

HUGGINS, C., MOON, R. C., MORRII, S.: Extinction of experimental mammary cancer. I. Estradiol-17β and Progesterone. Proc. nat. Acad. Sci. (Wash.) 48, 379 (1962).

JANTET, G., CROCKER, D. W., MASANORI, S., MORRE, F. D.: Adrenal suppression in disseminated carcinoma of the breast. I. The effect on adrenal morphology of hypophysectomy and corticosteroid treatment. New Engl. J. Med. 269, 1 (1963).

KENNEDY, B. J.: Hormone therapy for advanced breast cancer. Cancer 18, 1551 (1965).

LANDAU, R. L.: Can endocrine therapy be expected to replace the surgical treatment of advanced breast cancer? In: Major endocrine surgery for the treatment of cancer of the breast in advanced stages. Eds.: M. DARGENT and C. I. ROMIEU. Lyon: Simep édition 1967, p. 263.

— EHRLICH, E. N., HUGGINS, C.: Estradiol benzoate and progesterone in advanced human breast cancer. J. Amer. med. Ass. 182, 622 (1962).

LEMON, H. M.: Prednisone therapy in advanced mammary cancer. Cancer 12, 93 (1959).

NISSEN-MEYER, R., VOGT, J. H.: Five years' experience of the treatment of metastatic breast cancer. Mem. Soc. Endocr. 10, 124 (1961).

SEGALOFF, A., CARABASI, R., HORWITT, B. N., SCHLOSSER, J. V., MURISON, P. J.: Hormonal therapy in cancer of the breast. VI. Effect of ACTH and cortisone on clinical course and hormonal excretion. Cancer 71, 331 (1954).

SLAUNWHITE, N. R., SANDBERG, A. A.: Metabolism of 1-dehydro-17-hydroxy corticosteroids in human subjects. J. clin. Endocr. 17, 395 (1957).

STOLL, B. A.: Effect of Lyndiol, an oral contraceptive, on breast cancer. Brit. med. J. 1967 I, p. 150.

— ANDREWS, J. T., MOTTERAM, R.: Liver damage from oral contraceptives. Brit. med. J. 1966 I, p. 960.

Chapter 7

Antecedent and Racial Factors

A comparison between the histories of patients with breast cancer and of normal controls has resulted in the detection of certain features which breast cancer patients have in common. These features are mainly concerned with marital status and fertility and have appropriately been termed antecedent factors.

Recognition of these antecedent factors is important, because they are probably linked with changes in endocrine status and it may be these endocrine changes which play a part in the development of the disease. Investigation of such relationships is not easy. Although the epidemiological aspects of breast cancer have been extensively explored, there has been little progress in demonstrating an association between the antecedent factors and possible changes in hormone excretion. This may in part be due to a lack of information on normal levels of hormone excretion and this in its turn may reflect the need for more research into the methodology of hormone measurement. Moreover the associations between these antecedent factors and breast cancer development, although not trivial, are probably not sufficient to persuade clinicians to give practical advice to their patients. Those interested in cancer prevention and control may be able to advise patients to stop smoking to avoid carcinoma of the lung, but it is more difficult to encourage a woman to marry or to have a large family in order to diminish her chances of developing breast cancer. Nevertheless, recognition of these factors may stimulate further investigation into the associated changes in the hormonal environment and may indicate future paths for epidemiological research.

1. Heredity

Breast cancer is so common, that inevitably families will be encountered in which several members have developed the disease. Recently it has been recognised that this is a more frequent phenomenon than would be expected from a chance distribution. Retrospective studies have shown that in families of patients suffering from breast cancer there is approximately a two-fold excess of the disease amongst mothers and sisters (LILIENFELD, 1963), although from the available data it does not appear that a similar relationship exists with other close relatives such as aunts and grand-mothers (WYNDER, BROSS and HIRAYAMA, 1960).

There are several possible explanations for this finding. Members of these families have a similar environmental background, and certain social factors have been shown to correlate with the incidence of breast cancer (GRAHAM, LEVIN and LILIENFELD, 1960). A case can also be put forward for the existence of an agent which can be transmitted from mother to daughter. BITTNER (1937) described a virus-like particle in the milk of mice which he believed to be responsible for the transmission of a susceptibility to breast cancer. Similar particles have been demonstrated in human milk (PASSEY et al., 1951; GROSS, McCARTY and GESSLER, 1952) but there is little evidence relating their presence with the subsequent development of breast cancer. SYKES et al. (1968), in an electron microscopic study of human breast cancer, were unable to demonstrate intracellular structures resembling infectious or oncogenic viruses.

Few studies have been carried out to determine the extent to which patients with mammary cancer were breast fed, although the available evidence suggests that there is no relationship between incidence and maternal feeding in infancy (WYNDER et al., 1960). But memories are short—and few women know for certain if they were nursed at their mothers' breasts. ATKINS has tackled this problem in a forward study which he started in 1949. He has collected a panel of female infants known never to have had maternal milk and matched them with a control panel of infants breast fed in the normal way. He hopes it may be possible in the future to compare the incidence of breast cancer in these two groups (ATKINS, 1958).

On the other hand, the familial tendency to develop breast cancer may be a true inherited factor or—perhaps more likely—some other factor is inherited which in turn may be responsible for the development of the disease. Again there is little evidence of this. Studies have been carried out on breast cancer patients to see if they are predominantly of one blood group, but no correlation could be demonstrated (GOLDENBERG and HAYES, 1958; HARTMAN and STAVEN, 1964), although a similar investigation of gastric cancer patients had shown a significantly higher number than usual to be in Blood Group A (AIRD et al., 1955). One possibility is that a woman's basic pattern of hormone levels could be inherited and indeed it seems likely that this should be so; unfortunately few data are available on this but the inheritance of an abnormal endocrine environment could account for the high tendency to breast cancer noted in some families.

2. Marriage

Breast cancer is commoner in single than in married women. This is a consistent observation and the incidence of breast cancer in unmarried women and married controls has been reported by various investigators as 14.2 per cent and 5.9 per cent. (WAINWRIGHT, 1939) 6.6 per cent and 3.9 per cent (LEWISON and ALLEN, 1953) and 10.4 per cent and 7.1 per cent (WYNDER et al., 1960). It has also been noted that women who develop breast cancer married later than control patients and, possibly as a result of this, their first pregnancy tends to be later (LILIENFELD, 1961). LILIENFELD (1963) has reported an interesting association between marital status and the incidence of artificial menopause. In a study of the menopausal histories of patients admitted to the Roswell Park Memorial Institute in Buffalo he showed that the frequency of artificial menopause was 30 per cent less in single than in married women. Similarly the artificial menopause, which on average was 10 years earlier than the natural menopause, was less frequent in patients with breast cancer than in patients with cancers of other sites. He interpreted this as indicating that an artificial menopause may protect against breast cancer and that the difference in incidence of breast cancer in single and married women may simply reflect the incidence of artificial menopause. STOCKS (1958) however has shown that, although the death rate from breast cancer is less in married than in single women, the rates for infertile married women do not differ appreciably from those for single women.

3. Pregnancy and Parity

Although in most cases pregnancy will increase the rapidity of growth of existing tumours of the breast there is no evidence that it can stimulate breast cancer to develop. Indeed if anything, there is evidence to the contrary (BROOKS and PROFFITT, 1949). LANE-CLAYPON (1926) in her survey of antecedent factors in cancer of the breast noted a greater frequency of the disease in women who had never been pregnant, and it has also been shown to have an increased incidence amongst nuns (GAGNON, 1950). PELLER (1940) noted that breast cancer occurred more often in women having one pregnancy than in multipara and suggested that the incidence was inversely proportional to the number of children borne. Elsewhere LEWISON and ALLEN (1953) have reported that the average number of pregnancies per fertile women was 1.91 fewer in their cancer patients than in controls. WYNDER et al. (1960) however reported that a similar number of both breast cancer and control patients were nulliparous; they also noted no difference in the number having had abortions and, although a somewhat greater total number of pregnancies was found in the control group, this difference disappeared when the data were standardised for age at first pregnancy. LOGAN (1953) when analysing mortality rates, indicated that in patients over 35 years of age, mortality was higher from breast cancer among single women than among fertile women. However, in women under 35 years of age the opposite was the case and the greater number of deaths occurred in those who had borne children. This work has been criticised (LILIENFELD, 1963) because the death rates were based on a small number of cases.

To summarise, it seems likely that childbearing is protective against breast cancer although under what circumstances and to what degree is unknown. STOCKS (1958) may be correct in his interpretation of the British Empire Cancer Campaign's Merseyside survey. He believes that it is a dearth of confinements during the first ten years of the potential childbearing period which correlates with the increased risk of breast cancer over the age of 45, but if marriage is delayed then the number of confinements is unimportant. EISENBERG (1968) has made an important observation from data obtained from the Connecticut Tumour Registry. He has noticed that the menarche is now occurring at an earlier age in young girls. At the same time, women seem to be older when they have their first child. This means that a girl is menstruating but nulliparous for a longer time and EISENBERG believes that this may account for the recent increase in the incidence of breast cancer in young women.

4. Lactation

The relationship between lactation and breast cancer is similar to the relationship between pregnancy and breast cancer. Although the rate of growth seems enhanced if a tumour occurs in a lactating breast, lactation may be protective against a subsequent carcinoma. LILIENFELD (1963) discusses the relationship from three aspects: (a) The percentage of patients who have never breast fed their children, (b) the percentage of children who have never been breast fed, (c) the duration of breast feeding. He reviews the literature on the first two of these and finds the evidence conflicting in properly controlled studies. LANE-CLAYPON (1926) studied the history of breast feeding in 500 cancer patients and 500 controls; twice as many of the children of the cancer patients had not been fed at the breast.

Other controlled series, including as many cases, could not confirm this (WAINWRIGHT, 1931; MACMAHON and FEINLEIB, 1960). Similar confusion occurs when duration of lactation is considered. In a Japanese report, breast cancer patients over 45 years of age were shown to have breast fed their children for a shorter period of time than controls (KAMOI, 1960) but a similar correlation could not be demonstrated for breast cancer patients aged 35—44 nor for other racial groups (WYNDER et al., 1960; MACMAHON and FEINLEIB, 1960). It would certainly seem that if nursing plays any protective role in the incidence and development of breast cancer more definite evidence would by now be forthcoming. In the United States, breast feeding is relatively uncommon and yet the incidence of breast cancer amongst both negroes and whites is no higher than for most European countries. Similarly the habits of breast feeding for the urban Japanese have changed considerably both in duration and extent over the last 20 years but there is no sign as yet of an increase in the incidence of breast disease. It has been suggested that any slight protection that may result from lactation may be due to the secondary hormone effects rather than from any direct local changes—for instance, during the nursing period ovarian function is diminished (LILIENFELD, 1963). If this influences the development of breast cancer, the effect must be very slight.

5. Menstrual History and the Menopause

It does not appear that vagaries of menstruation have any effect on the development of breast cancer. Comparisons between the incidence of the disease and such factors as duration of loss, duration of cycle or menstrual abnormalities have not shown any correlation (WYNDER et al., 1960; MACMAHON and FEINLEIB, 1960). During the first four decades the incidence of breast cancer increases with age, but over 45 this increase in incidence lessens and it has been postulated that the percentage of women in the population who are susceptible to the disease diminishes. Also after this age the difference in incidence rates between single and married women becomes more apparent (KAMOI, 1960). This change in incidence at about the time of the menopause has frequently been reported and was originally described by CLEMMENSEN (1948). As a result it has been argued that the menopause is to an extent protective and that the earlier it occurs, the less likelihood there is of a woman developing cancer of the breast. Certainly, the mean age at the menopause of postmenopausal cancer patients is slightly greater than that of controls (OLCH, 1937) and this difference is significant (MACMAHON and FEINLEIB, 1960). It has also been shown that the incidence of early artificial menopause is lower in breast cancer patients (LILIENFELD, 1956; MACMAHON and FEINLEIB, 1960) than in controls. DE WAARD et al. (1960) have accounted for these changes in incidence during the fifth decade by postulating that the population of mammary cancer patients in Western countries is composed of two populations each having its own age distribution and having their highest frequencies of tumour production at 45 and 65 years of age. They further propose that the disease may result from ovarian disfunction in the younger group and adrenal disfunction in the older. They provide data to show that more postmenopausal breast cancer patients suffer from obesity and hypertension than a control group and that this might result from adrenal oestrogenic activity.

6. Bilateral Disease

If breast cancer may result from an abnormality of endogenous hormone production then all breast tissue will be affected by the abnormal environment and be equally at risk. As the abnormality will probably continue after a mastectomy these patients should stand a greater than normal chance of developing a second primary carcinoma in the opposite breast. Confusion can occur here in determining whether a tumour developing on the opposite side is a new primary or a metastasis from the original lesion. There is no simple method of distinction, but a combination of rigid clinical and pathological criteria such as described by ROBBINS and BERG (1964) probably does not allow for much error. In a prospective study of 1,458 patients with breast cancer they described 94 patients who subsequently developed bilateral disease. They assessed this as representing 7 cases per year ten thousand patients at risk which is approximately five times the incidence in the general female population. This finding agrees with data reported by other workers (MIDER et al., 1952; HUBBARD, 1953). When the incidence in patients under 50 years of age was assessed this figure rose to ten times the normal. The incidence is most common in patients who have multiple cancers in the first breast giving further indication perhaps to some generalised extra-mammary stimulation.

Furthermore, because these women have had one breast removed, the amount of breast tissue at risk for developing a further primary carcinoma is reduced by half, and one would therefore expect that the incidence of new primaries would also be half that of the general female population. On this basis the reported rate of five times the normal might be more accurately expressed as ten times the normal and the incidence in patients under 50 as twenty times the normal.

Even allowing for some error in distinguishing between a metastasis and a new primary, this increased liability is of the greatest significance. The breast cancer patients who have abnormalities of hormone excretion at the time of mastectomy (BULBROOK et al., 1962) may be those who stand the risk of developing a second primary. If this is so then a correction of this abnormality might lead to a reduction in the number of patients who will suffer from bilateral disease.

7. Gynaecological Disease

Many studies have been attempted to investigate the subsequent development of breast cancer in patients with gynaecological disease. In view of the recognised beneficial effect that can result from oophorectomy in advanced breast cancer and also its possible value as a prophylactic measure in the early disease, women who have had their ovaries removed for other reasons might stand a less than normal chance of developing breast cancer. Indeed some reports in the literature have shown this to be so (LILIENFELD, 1963; MacMAHON and FEINLEIB, 1960; HIRAYAMA and WYNDER, 1962) but others have hinted that the opposite may occur (SWERDLOW and HUMPHREY, 1964) and the question remains open. There is also a suggestion that if castrated women develop breast cancer more than one year after the operation then the prognosis tends to be poor (SWERDLOW and HUMPHREY, 1964; DARGENT, 1949).

Taken as a whole, the over-all incidence of gynaecological disease and gynaecological operations is not greater in breast cancer patients than in patients with benign breast disease or controls (LEWISON and ALLEN, 1953). On the other hand certain cancers of the genital tract seem more closely related, and in two large series the incidence of cancer of the body of the uterus has been reported to vary directly with the incidence of breast cancer (WYNDER et al., 1960; BAILAR, 1963). The probable reason for this is that both diseases occur in the same type of patient—for instance both are commoner in single women. A similar but negative correlation can be shown between breast cancer and cancer of the uterine cervix, a disease which is predominant in married women. Indeed in one series there were more breast cancer patients subsequently developing fundal than cervical primaries, a distribution which is opposite to that in the general population (WYNDER et al., 1960).

Nevertheless, it seems unlikely that this association with both types of uterine neoplasms is more than a coincidental relationship. Both carcinoma of the uterus and carcinoma of the breast are probably influenced by similar predisposing factors.

Breast cancer has also been reported to be common in patients who have had salivary gland cancer. BERG et al. (1968) reported that the subsequent incidence of breast cancer in 396 patients with known cancers of the major salivary glands was eight times the normal. The reason for this association is obscure.

8. Racial Factors

The possible importance of racial factors in the aetiology of breast cancer has only recently been investigated. It had been known for a long time that certain races have a high incidence of the disease whilst others have a very low incidence. Exact figures are very difficult to obtain because the system of reporting is inadequate in many countries. Cancer is seldom made a notifiable disease and it is only in very restricted areas, such as the State of Connecticut in the United States of America, that accurate figures of incidence have been recorded for any length of time. A reasonable compromise has been to make use of death rates. These are more often recorded than incidence rates, although again in many underdeveloped countries the medical and administrative facilities make the accurate recording of death rates almost impossible.

SEGI (1957) listed the death rates per 100,000 population in many countries, and data from his work have been the basis for many investigations. Fig. 14 is based on SEGI's figures and lists the death rates in ten countries. The most remarkable is between the rates in most Western countries and the rates in Japan—for instance, the disease is about eight times commoner in England and Wales than in Japan.

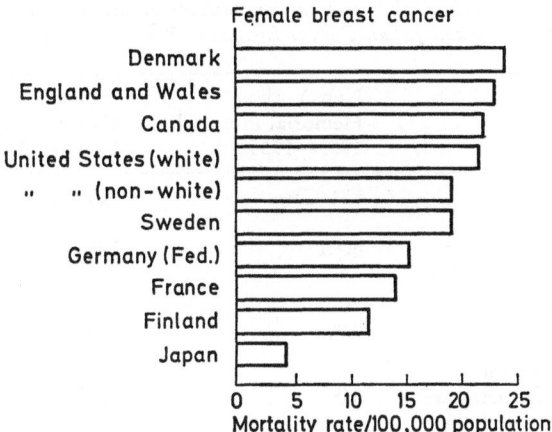

Fig. 14. The mortality rate from breast cancer in various countries. Female breast cancer. (From SEGI, 1957)

This low incidence of breast cancer is not a feature common to Oriental countries but more specifically typical of the Japanese race. WYNDER et al. (1960) remark that the Chinese do not have a similar low incidence of breast cancer, although the data in this respect are rather suspect and BUELL (1965) has since given the mortality rate from breast cancer of Chinese residents in California as being 6.8 per 100,000, compared with 5.3 per 100,000 for Japanese residents and 27.6 per 100,000 for the white population. On the other hand, KOUWENAAR (1950—1951) noted that of the histologically proven cancers in Chinese women, breast cancer accounted for 23 per cent—a percentage very similar to that found in the West. Similarly, VELLIOS (1955) found breast cancer to be common in Thailand.

Some other countries also have a low incidence. The reported deaths from breast cancer in Chile indicate a rate not much greater than that found in Japan (MAISIN and LANGEROCK, 1955). Also breast cancer is rare in Finland, compared with the rates in neighbouring Scandinavian countries. Denmark, has the highest death rate from breast cancer in the world.

There also seems to be some evidence that the behaviour of breast tumours in Japanese women differs from the behaviour of tumours in women from countries where the disease is more common. WYNDER et al. (1963) compared patients with operable breast cancer at the Japan Cancer Institute in Tokyo with similar patients at the Memorial Hospital in New York. They found that the five year survival rate of all patients with primary operable breast cancer was 74 per cent in Tokyo, compared with 60 per cent in New York. Also 51 per cent of the Japanese patients who were operated on had no metastases in the axillary lymph nodes, compared with 43 per cent of the Americans. Table 21 summarises the main features of this comparison. There are, of course, many pitfalls in making a retrospective comparison of survival rates between patients in different hospitals and in different countries, but WYNDER and his colleagues believe that the improved survival in Japan could not be accounted for by differences in age, size of primary lesion, histology of the tumour or therapy. They comment that the patients treated at the Japanese Cancer

Table 21. *Comparison of survival of breast cancer patients admitted to the Memorial Hospital, New York and Japan Cancer Institute.* (WYNDER et al., 1963)

	New York Memorial Hospital 1953—1955	Japan Cancer Institute 1946—1955
	581 Cases	401 Cases
5-year survival of all primary operable breast cancer	60%	74%
Stage 1	79%	88%
Stage 2	46%	59%
Percentage with lymph node metastases at time of mastectomy	51%	43%

Institute were more selected but, when the comparison was made taking the stage of the disease into account (Table 21), there was still a difference in survival in each stage. It seems unlikely that selection could have played much part in affecting the survival within each stage. Also the Japanese cases included nineteen patients in whom the supraclavicular nodes were involved. These patients would not have been considered operable by the Memorial Hospital in New York, and their inclusion would tend to make the Japanese survival figures worse.

WYNDER and his colleagues suggested that an explanation of these findings might lie in an endocrine difference in American and Japanese women which not only decreased the risk of Japanese women developing breast cancer but also increased their survival expectancy if they developed the disease. They concluded ... "the present study may serve as an impetus to the steroid chemist to determine endocrine differences in these groups."

This suggestion was taken up by BULBROOK and his colleagues (1964). They collected a 24-hour urine specimen from twenty-four Japanese women living in Tokyo, and fifty-nine British women living in the United Kingdom. On the assumption that endogenous androgen levels might affect the incidence of breast cancer (see pp. 124—131 and also BULBROOK and HAYWARD, 1967), they compared the 11-deoxy-17-oxosteroid excretion of the Japanese and British women. The 11-deoxy-17-oxosteroids are products of androgen metabolism. Rather unexpectedly, the secretion of these steroids was significantly lower in Japanese women than in British women, although this difference disappeared when height and weight were taken into account and when the steroid measurements were expressed in terms of creatinine excretion. But BULBROOK et al. (1964) found one further difference in androgen excretion which could not be accounted for by differences in stature between the two races. The 11-deoxy-17-oxosteroids are composed of three compounds, aetiocholanolone, androsterone and dehydroepiandrosterone. Androsterone has some androgenic activity (0.1 mg androsterone $\equiv$ 100 I. U. androgenic activity—Comb Growth Test), whereas aetiocholanolone has none. Structurally androsterone and aetiocholanolone are identical except that in androsterone the hydrogen atom on the fith carbon atom is in the alpha position whereas in aetiocholanolone it is in the beta position.

The quantitative relationship of androsterone to aetiocholanolone is known as the $5\alpha/5\beta$ ratio. BULBROOK and his colleagues found the mean $5\alpha/5\beta$ ratio to be 1.3 in the twenty-four Japanese women, whereas it was only 1.0 in the British controls. The difference in the ratios was statistically significant. There is no information on whether this difference in the $5\alpha/5\beta$ ratio has any bearing on the different incidence of breast cancer in Japanese and British women. But it seems that Japanese women metabolise their androgens in a different way from British women, so that more is excreted as androsterone which is the more active compound. In view of the evidence that androgen excretion in British women is markedly correlated with the incidence and prognosis of breast cancer (see pages 124—131 and 80—82), this difference in the $5\alpha/5\beta$ ratio in the Japanese and British women could be of fundamental importance in the understanding of the difference in the behaviour of the disease between the two races. BULBROOK and his colleagues remark that the $5\alpha/5\beta$ ratio tends to be higher in hyperthyroid patients and have questioned whether the high values found in Japanese women indicate a greater degree of thyroid activity. Thyroid function again has a bearing on the incidence of breast cancer in that the disease is probably more common in hypothyroid women (see pages 140—141).

In a subsequent report, BULBROOK et al. (1967) compared the excretion of the urinary 17-OHCS and the 11-deoxy-17-oxosteroids in thirty-three Japanese women with that in forty-one British women. When the determinations were corrected for weight, it was found that in young women, the British excreted more of these compounds than the Japanese. In older women, the situation was reversed and the Japanese aged over fifty-five excreted more 11-deoxy-17-oxosteroids than British women over fifty-five.

BULBROOK and his colleagues (1967) were also able to confirm their previous observations on the differences in the $5\alpha/5\beta$ ratio between the British and Japanese women. The Japanese women had a mean $5\alpha/5\beta$ ratio of 1.304, whereas in the British women, the mean ratio was 0.994; the difference between the means was again significant.

They further analysed their subjects by age groups and found that the main differences in the $5\alpha/5\beta$ ratio were in the groups 40—59 and 50—59. The differences in the ratio in patients aged between 20 and 29 were minimal (see Fig. 15). The differences in the mortality rates from breast cancer between British and Japanese women also do not become marked until the age of forty-five (see BUELL, 1965). In the younger age groups, the mortality per 100,000 population is very similar. However, BULBROOK and his colleagues (1967) caution that their results lend no support to the thesis that the low incidence of breast cancer in Japanese women would be due to high levels of endogenous hormones.

The incidence of breast cancer in immigrant populations has been studied to see whether the rate remains that of the country of origin or becomes the same as the country of adoption. There is a big immigrant Japanese population in Hawaii and their incidence of breast cancer per 100,000 has been calculated from the admissions to the Queen's Hospital in Honolulu (SMITH, 1956). The incidence rate for white women was 33.5 per 100,000 whilst that for Japanese women was 7.1—a difference similar to that noted between the populations of the United States of America and Japan. BUELL (1965) reviewed the cancer mortality rates in California in whites, negroes, Chinese, Japanese and Phillipinos. Here again, there is a high immigrant

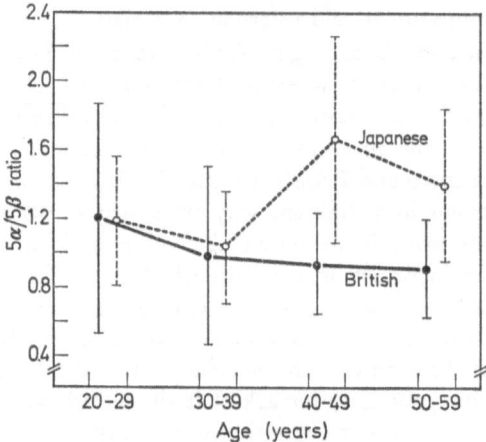

Fig. 15. Comparison of ratio of androsterone: aetiocholanolone in normal British and Japanese women in four age groups. The vertical bars represent the range of the 5a : 5β ratio. (From BULBROOK et al., 1967; reproduced with permission)

Japanese population (79,750 in 1960) who seem to maintain a cancer rate similar to that of their country of origin. The rate per 100,000 in the immigrant Japanese was 5.3 compared with 27.6 for the local white population.

There is some evidence that when Japanese are born in their country of adoption, as opposed to being first generation immigrants, their cancer mortality rate changes. Although the characteristic pattern of difference is retained, the degree of difference becomes less. This may indicate that the typically high or low incidence of certain cancers in Japan is more likely to be environmental in origin than genetic. BUELL and DUNN (1965) have compared the cancer mortality rate of Japanese Issei (first generation or immigrant generation) and Nisei (second generation) in California. They have shown that, for each succeeding generation in the immigrant Japanese, there is a tendency for the mortality rate from cancer—particularly from tumours of the stomach—to come nearer the mortality rate of the native white American. This tendency was shown in the breast cancer rate, although the numbers were small. Taking the California rate for whites to be 1.0, the native Japanese rate was 0.2 and that for the Japanese Nisei in California was 0.3. A more recent study by HAENSZEL and KURIHARA (1968) has not confirmed this tendency. They studied the cancer mortality among U.S. Issei and Nisei Japanese for 1959—1962. Although the mortality rates for some cancers (particularly colon) had changed to that of U.S. white, there was no tendency for the breast cancer rate to rise to the level of the host population.

If the mortality rate from cancer of the breast in immigrant Japanese is eventually going to approximate to that of the native white population, it is important to investigate the reason for this. There are many changes that occur in the life and environment of these immigrants and it is difficult to single out the factor or factors which influence the development of cancer of the breast. The more obvious changes, like breast feeding habits, which are believed marginally to influence the incidence of breast cancer (see page 102), do not appear to have any effect. The breast cancer rate in the United States of America has not altered to any extent over the past thirty years, although fewer American women now feed their children at the breast. There is also evidence that the low incidence of breast cancer in Japan occurs in both males and females (LILIENFELD, 1963). This would be unlikely if breast feeding habits were a reasonable explanation of the low breast cancer mortality in Japan.

Apart from climate, which may itself have an influence on the development of breast cancer (see LEA, 1965), the most obvious environmental change to Japanese immigrants may be their diet. WYNDER and HOFFMAN (1967) suggest that any increase in the incidence rate of breast cancer in Japanese immigrants in California and Hawaii may in part be due to changes in basic nutrition. They note that the average fat consumption of Japanese in Japan is approximately 10 per cent of the total caloric intake and is mostly unsaturated fat, whereas in the United States of America, the fat consumption is over 40 per cent of the total caloric intake and is mostly in the saturated form. They suggest that food intake and the secretion of endogenous hormones may be correlated. BULBROOK and his colleagues (1966) are investigating this hypothesis by measuring the hormone excretion of Japanese immigrants to Vancouver. Like the west coast of the United States of America, Vancouver has a big Japanese immigrant population. Since the original immigrant families settled in Canada, several generations have been born, and with each generation the way of life has become more Westernised. This is particularly marked in their dietary habits. First generation Japanese will eat mostly Japanese food, whereas when the second or third generations are reached the diet of the immigrant families becomes very similar to that of the Canadians. BULBROOK and his co-workers are measuring the excretion of the 11-deoxy-17-oxosteroids in these Japanese families and comparing the urinary levels of these compounds with the Westernisation of the diet. In particular, they are examining the value of the $5\alpha/5\beta$ ratio to see if this becomes nearer unity, and hence nearer to the British values, as the diets of these immigrants change. No results of this work are available.

The measurement of endogenous hormone levels in native and immigrant populations is a completely new and largely unexplored field of investigation. In view of the large racial differences in the incidence of breast cancer and the mounting evidence of the part that hormones may play in aetiology, further research is essential in this subject. Unfortunately, the assessment of endogenous hormone levels is bedevilled with many hazards. Apart from the methodological difficulties, many of which have still to be overcome, there is the almost insuperable problem of the variations in hormone levels which may result from extraneous influences. Some of the reasons for these variations are known and can be allowed for, but many are unknown and may have an incalculable effect on the accuracy of urinary hormone measurements. BULBROOK (1966) touched on this problem in discussing the measurement of the hormonal status and, apart from within-subject variability, he listed age, weight, drugs, stress and illness as being potent causes of changes in hormone excretion. Almost certainly, there are many more, each of which could bias a population study in an unpredictable way.

Summary and Conclusions

1. The incidence of breast cancer is commoner in women whose mothers or sisters have had the disease.

2. Marriage, pregnancy and possibly lactation are protective.

3. Women who have had cancer in one breast are more susceptible to develop a second primary in the opposite breast.

4. The incidence of breast cancer is decreased in women who have had an early artificial menopause.

5. Cancer of the body of the uterus and cancer of the breast occur in the same women more often than would be expected by chance.

6. Cancer of the uterine cervix and breast rarely occur together.

7. Breast cancer is commoner in Western countries than in the Orient.

8. There is a particularly low incidence in Japan where the disease also runs a more benign course.

9. There is mounting evidence that all the above correlations may be endocrine based.

References

AIRD, I., DICKINS, A. M., RICHARDSON, J. R. E., ROBERTS, J. A. F.: Discussion on ABO blood groups and disease. Proc. roy. Soc. Med. 48, 139 (1955).

ATKINS, H. J. B.: A study in the transmission of maternal antibodies. Brit. med. J. 1958 I, 187.

BAILAR, J. C.: The incidence of independent tumours among uterine cancer patients. Cancer 16, 842 (1963).

BERG, J. W., HUTTER, R. V. P., FOOTE, F. W.: The unique association between salivary gland cancer and breast cancer. J. Amer. med. Ass. 204, 113 (1968).

BITTNER, J. J.: Some possible effects of nursing on the mammary gland tumour incidence in mice. Science 84, 162 (1936).

BROOKS, B., PROFFITT, J. N.: The influence of pregnancy on cancer of the breast. Surgery 25, 1 (1949).

BUELL, P.: Cancer mortality of selected sites in racial groups of California. Chronic Disease Quarterly (Suppl.) 6 (1965).

— DUNN, J. E.: Cancer mortality among Japanese Issei and Nisei of California. Cancer 18, 656 (1965).

BULBROOK, R. D.: Measurement of hormonal status. In: Clinical Evaluation in Breast Cancer. Eds.: J. L. HAYWARD and R. D. BULBROOK. London-New York: Academic Press 1966, p. 77.

— HAMAGUCHI, E., MACDONALD, W. C., THOMAS, B. S., UTSUNOMIYA, J.: Urinary 11-deoxy-17-oxosteroid and 17-hydroxycorticosteroid excretion in British women living in Tokyo and Vancouver in relation to the incidence of breast cancer. Abstracts Ninth Int. Cancer Congress 1966, p. 653.

— HAYWARD, J. L.: Abnormal urinary steroid excretion and subsequent breast cancer. Lancet 1967 I, 519.

— — SPICER, C. C., THOMAS, B. S.: Abnormal excretion of urinary steroids by women with early breast cancer. Lancet 1962 II, 1238.

— THOMAS, B. S., UTSUNOMIYA, J., HAMAGUCHI, E.: The urinary excretion of 11-deoxy-17-oxosteroids and 17-hydroxycorticosteroids by normal Japanese and British women. J. Endocr. 38, 401 (1967).

— — — Urinary 11-deoxy-17-oxosteroids in British and Japanese women with reference to the incidence of breast cancer. Nature 201, 189 (1964).

CLEMMENSEN, J.: Carcinoma of breast; symposium; results from statistical research. Brit. J. Radiol. 21, 583 (1948).

DARGENT, M.: Carcinoma of the breast in castrated women. Brit. med. J. 1949 II, 54.

DEWAARD, R., DELAIVE, J. W. J., BAANDERS VAN HALEWIJN, E. A.: On the bimodal age distribution of mammary carcinoma. Brit. J. Cancer 14, 437 (1960).

EISENBERG, H.: Personal Communication 1968.

GAGNON, F.: Contribution to study of etiology and prevention of cancer of cervix of uterus. Amer. J. Obstet. Gynec. 60, 516 (1950).

GOLDENBERG, I. S., HAYES, M. A.: Breast carcinoma and ABO blood groups. Cancer 11, 973 (1958).

GRAHAM, S., LEVIN, M., LILIENFELD, A.: The socioeconomic distribution of cancer of various sites in Buffalo, N. Y. Cancer 13, 180 (1960).

GROSS, L., McCARTY, K. S., GESSLER, A. E.: The significance of particles in human milk. Ann. N. Y. Acad. Sci. 54, 1018 (1952).

HAENSZEL, N., KURIHARA, M.: Studies of Japanese migrants. I. Mortality from cancer and other diseases among Japanese in the United States. J. nat. Cancer Inst. 40, 43 (1968).

HARTMAN, D., STAVEM, P.: ABO blood groups and cancer. Lancet 1964 I, 1305.

HIRAYAMA, T., WYNDER, E. L.: A study of the epidemology of cancer of the breast. II. The influence of hysterectomy. Cancer 15, 28 (1962).

HUBBARD, T. B.: Nonsimultaneous bilateral carcinoma of the breast. Surgery 34, 706 (1953).

KAMOI, M.: Statistical study on relation between cancer and lactation period. I. A comparative study through cumulative frequency distribution. Tohoku J. exp. Med. 72, 72 (1960).

KOUWENAAR, W.: On cancer incidence in Indonesia. (Abstr.) J. nat. Cancer Inst. 11, 642 (1950—1951).

LANE-CLAYPON, J. E.: A further report on cancer of the breast, with special reference to its associated antecedent conditions. Public Health and Medical Subjects No. 32. London: British Ministry of Health 1926.

LEA, A. J.: New observations on distribution of neoplasms of female breast in certain European countries. Brit. med. J. 1965 I, 488.

LEWISON, E. F., ALLEN, L. W.: Antecedent factors in cancer of the breast. Ann. Surg. 138, 39 (1953).

LILIENFELD, A. M.: The relationship of cancer of the female breast to artificial menopause and marital status. Cancer 9, 927 (1956).

— Some epidemiologic aspects of cancer of the breast. Proceedings Fourth National Cancer Conference. Philadelphia: J. B. Lippincott Co. 1961, p. 215.

— The epidemiology of breast cancer. Cancer Res. 23, 1503 (1963).

LOGAN, W. P. D.: Marriage and childbearing in relation to cancer of the breast and uterus. Lancet 1953 II, 1199.

MacMAHON, B., FEINLEIB, M.: Breast cancer in relation to nursing and menopausal history. J. nat. Cancer Inst. 24, 733 (1960).

MAISIN, J. H., LANGEROCK, G.: Racial factors in the causation of carcinoma of the breast. Schweiz. Z. Path. 18, 690 (1955).

MIDER, G. B., SCHILLING, J. A., DONOVAN, J. C., RENDALL, E. S.: Multiple cancer. A study of other causes arising in patients with primary malignant neoplasms of the stomach, uterus, breast, large intestine or hematopoietic system. Cancer 5, 1105 (1952).

OLCH, I. Y.: Menopausal age in women with cancer of the breast. Amer. J. Cancer 30, 563 (1937).

PASSEY, R. D., DMOCHOWSKI, L., ASTBURY, W. T., REED, R., EAVES, G.: Electron microscope studies of human breast cancer. Nature 167, 643 (1951).

PELLER, S.: Cancer and it's relations to pregnancy, to delivery, and to marital and social status. I. Cancer of the breast and genital organs. Surg. Gynec. Obstet. 71, 1 (1940).

ROBBINS, G. F., BERG, J. W.: Bilateral primary breast cancer. A prospective clinicopathological study. Cancer 17, 1501 (1964).

SEGI, M.: Cancer mortality statistics in Japan 1953—1955. Sendai, Japan, Department of Public Health, Tohoku University 1957.

SMITH, R. L.: Recorded and expected mortality among Japanese of United States and Hawaii with special reference to cancer. J. nat. Cancer Inst. 17, 459 (1956).

STOCKS, P.: Statistical investigations concerning the causation of various forms of human cancer. In: Cancer, Vol. 3. Ed.: R. W. RAVEN. London: Butterworth 1958, p. 116.

SWERDLOW, M., HUMPHREY, L. G.: The relationship of breast disease to gynaecologic disease. Cancer 17, 1165 (1964).

SYKES, J. A., RECHER, L., JERNSTROM, P. H., WHITESCARVER, J.: Morphological investigation of human breast cancer. J. nat. Cancer Inst. 40, 195 (1968).

VELLIOS, F.: Tumours of breast; their occurrence in Thailand. Schweiz. Z. allg. Path. 18, 722 (1955).

WAINWRIGHT, J. H.: Comparison of conditions associated with breast cancer in Great Britain and America. Amer. J. Cancer 15, 2610 (1931).

WYNDER, E. L., BROSS, I. J., HIRAJAMA, T.: A study of the epidemiology of cancer of the breast. Cancer 13, 559 (1960).

— HOFFMAN, D.: Nutrition and Cancer. In: The prevention of cancer. Eds.: R. W. RAVEN and F. J. C. ROE. London: Butterworths 1967, p. 11.

— KAJITANI, T., KUNO, J., LUCAS, J. C., DE PALO, A., FARROW, J.: A comparison of survival rates between American and Japanese patients with breast cancer. Surg. Gynec. Obstet. 117, 196 (1963).

Chapter 8

Oestrogens

Breast cancer can be induced in some laboratory animals by the administration of oestrogens (see for instance LACCASSAGNE, 1932; SHIMKIN and WYMAN, 1946), but there is considerable variation in response and it cannot be inferred that oestrogens have the same effect in man. Naturally no experimental work has been undertaken to induce human breast cancer by this or any other means. Nevertheless, in man, prolonged oestrogen therapy or a pathological excess of naturally occurring hormones can result in similar conditions to those induced experimentally in animals. Such circumstances are rare. Oestrogens are seldom administered for long periods and marked increases in levels of the natural compounds occur only with feminising tumours or certain endocrine anomalies. The contraceptive pill contains small amounts of oestrogen and, in the future, its use may provide information on the results of long term administration. To date, the pill has not been available long enough to provide any meaningful evidence.

Exogenous Oestrogens

1. Males

Oestrogen administration can stimulate the development of breast carcinoma in male mice to the rate found normally in females of the same strain (see page 1). Therefore, the prolonged administration of oestrogen to man might be associated with an increase in the incidence of breast cancer to the rate found in women. Human male breast cancer is rare but when it occurs it has very similar histological and behavioural characteristics to the condition in the female. In the early stages it can be treated by radical mastectomy and, when advanced, may be amenable to hormone therapy, castration or hypophysectomy. In Western countries, it represents only 0.9 per cent of the female incidence and accounts for little more than 0.2 per cent of all male cancer. Thus any increase in incidence should be readily detected.

Oestrogens are commonly administered to treat carcinoma of the prostate. Here the beneficial effect can be considerable and so prolonged that the prescription of the drug is often continued for many years. Gynaecomastia is a frequent complication but only occasionally is the breast development so extensive to be an embarrassment to the patient. Soon after oestrogen therapy was first introduced, reports began to appear of patients developing carcinoma of the breast following treatment. LIEBEGOTT (1948), ENTZ (1948), and GRAVES and HARRIS (1952) all described malignant tumours of the breast occurring in men on oestrogen therapy, and ABRAMSON and

Warshawsky (1948), Howard and Grosjean (1949), Corbett and Abrams (1950), and Jakobsen (1952) similarly reported bilateral breast carcinomata developing in men after prolonged treatment.

There was difficulty in the interpretation of these reports and this difficulty was emphasised by many of the authors. These patients were being treated for carcinoma of the prostate, and this tumour can metastasise to the breast. Under these circumstances, the metastasis in the breast could easily be confused both clinically and histologically with a primary breast cancer. For instance, Entz (1948) believed his patient's breast tumour was a metastasis whereas the tumours described by Liebegott (1948) and Graves and Harris (1952), both had axillary metastases, and would seem more likely to be primary. Campbell and Cummins (1951) reviewed the literature on men who developed breast cancer whilst on oestrogen therapy and added a case of their own. The patient had widespread metastases from a prostatic carcinoma and also a tumour in the breast. By histochemical techniques, Campbell and Cummins showed that the breast tumour was a secondary deposit. Benson (1957) suggested that not only could it be difficult to distinguish histologically between primary breast tumours and secondary deposits from the prostate, but also that patients with prostatic cancer who were receiving oestrogens were more liable to develop metastases in the breast. He felt that the structural changes that occurred in the breast following oestrogen therapy rendered it a more favourable medium in which cancer cells could settle and multiply.

In 1951 McClure and Higgins reported on a carcinoma of the breast which developed in a man treated with oestrogens for carcinoma of the bladder and it seemed unlikely that confusion could have occurred here; this patient also had a strong family history of breast cancer on the female side. But in a later report McClure (1951) stated that the autopsy findings revealed the bladder and breast tumours to be indistinguishable histologically. On the other hand, in 1953 Baierl described a carcinoma of the breast occurring in a 52 year old man under treatment with oestrogens for a peptic ulcer; a mastectomy was carried out and no other primary cancer was ever found.

Although there are many reports of male breast cancer occurring during oestrogen treatment, little is known about the size of the population at risk. Jakobsen (1952) commented that no breast carcinoma has been reported in a man with prostatic cancer who was not on oestrogen therapy. But this statement has since been challenged. Benson (1965) described a correspondence between Gaspari and Gardini (1948) in which three male patients were mentioned who had coexistent breast and prostatic cancers but were not on oestrogen therapy. Benson also remarked that Guthorn (1951), Hertz (1951) and Treves and Holleb (1955) each reported one case of such an association.

At the moment the situation seems confused and reports of individual cases have done little to further our understanding of the problem. Nevertheless the principle of whether administered oestrogens can cause breast cancer in man is an important one, and a prospective trial on the issue would be well worthwhile. It is probable that prolonged oestrogen administration does effect an increase in the incidence of male breast cancer but it is doubtful whether this increased incidence is sufficient to influence the decision whether to prescribe oestrogen for prostatic cancer—in itself a lethal disease.

Nevertheless some caution should be exercised when using oestrogen therapy to treat innocent conditions. SYMMERS (1968) related the remarkable history of two transvestite males who underwent complicated surgical operations to change their appearance to that of women. These operations included amputation of the penis, castration, bilateral mammoplasty and in one case the formation of a pro vagina using a length of bowel. For a long period the men took oestrogens by mouth, implant and breast inunction; one of the men even took the contraceptive pill for a while. Each developed a breast carcinoma which, in spite of radical mastectomy, eventually caused his death.

2. Females

At least one in every 25 female infants born will develop breast cancer during her adult life. This high incidence makes the chance that a tumour may develop whilst she is coincidentally receiving oestrogen therapy very considerable. It also makes an attempt to correlate oestrogen therapy with the incidence of breast cancer more difficult. Moreover, until the introduction of the contraceptive pill, it was unusual for women to be treated with hormones for a long period except perhaps occasionally for menopausal symptoms.

Some evidence that oestrogen therapy does not produce much structural change in the breast was provided by FOOTE and STEWART (1945). They compared the histological appearance of breasts in women having prolonged oestrogen treatment with the appearance in those who had not taken the drug. FOOTE and STEWART concluded there was little if any difference and, in reporting 4 cases of breast cancer in women who had been on oestrogen therapy, were unable to find any association between taking the drug and the development of the tumour. ALLABEN and OWEN (1939), AUCHINLOSS and HAAGENSEN (1940) and PARSONS and McCALL (1941) each reported on a case occurring in a woman during prolonged oestrogen treatment but on no occasion could the association be considered proven. On the other hand WAGGONER (1948), in describing a further case, went on to report on 31 other female patients with breast cancer in whom he considered there was some evidence of endocrine abnormality.

WILSON (1962) described a personal series of 304 female patients who for various reasons had received prolonged oestrogen therapy to a total of 2,387 patient years. He found no cancer of either breast or uterus in this group although he estimated that 18 cases should have occurred. As a result of this he postulated that oestrogens may be prophylactic against mammary and genital cancer.

These various reports lend little support to the thesis that prolonged oestrogen therapy can be carcinogenic. In women, there is as yet no direct evidence of a cause and effect relationship between oestrogen administration and the development of breast cancer.

Endogenous Oestrogens

1. Males

Little is known of any relationship between abnormal endocrine hormone production and the development of male breast cancer. Few data are available on the oestrogen excretion of normal men and men with breast cancer, although such a comparison might be interesting. The measurement of basic levels of excretion would possibly have more meaning in men than in women because there would be no variation due to a menstrual cycle.

Some studies have been carried out on the metabolism of administered hormones. ZUMOFF et al. (1966) administered oestradiol to men with breast cancer, and to control groups of normal men and men with other malignant disease. Intravenous injections of radioactive oestradiol were given and the excretion of 2-hydroxyoestrone, 2-methoxyoestrone, oestrone, oestradiol and oestriol was measured in a three day pool of urine. The excretion of oestradiol was similar in the three groups but the men with breast cancer excreted considerably less 2-hydroxyoestrone, 2-methoxy-oestrone, and oestrone, and much higher amounts of oestriol than the controls. In two patients these findings were not altered by subsequent castration. ZUMOFF and his colleagues considered that their results implied a relationship between oestrogen biotransformation and male breast cancer. They also believed their findings were encouraging in the search for endogenous factors that might be operative in the disease.

LILIENFELD (1963), in a study of male breast cancer, noted some association with conditions in which hormone levels might be disturbed. Twenty two per cent of 53 males with breast cancer gave a history of either orchitis, orchidectomy, therapeutic X-ray exposure or benign breast disease. In 53 matched controls with colonic cancer only 2 per cent had a history of these characteristics. He interpreted these data as suggesting that the influence of hormonal factor is important in the aetiology of breast cancer but suggested that more definitive and precise studies were needed.

JACKSON et al. (1965) investigated the occurrence of the Klinefelter syndrome in men with breast cancer. They described three cases of the Klinefelter syndrome occurring in 21 men suffering from carcinoma of the breast, whilst the normal incidence of the Klinefelter syndrome is less than 1 in 400. JACKSON and his colleagues estimated that the incidence of breast cancer in Klinefelter males approaches that of the normal female population.

Although the Klinefelter syndrome may be associated with gynaecomastia and hypogonadism, oestrogen levels do not appear to be raised and are variously reported as normal or below normal (HELLER and NELSON, 1944; GIORGI and SOMMER-VILLE, 1963). Gonadotrophin levels are frequently raised but 17-oxosteroid excretion tends to be low and an analogy can be drawn with the low androgen excretion found in many female patients with breast cancer (see page 123).

2. Females

In theory, if the incidence of breast cancer in women was affected by abnormal endogenous oestrogen production this could be determined by direct measurement. Methods are now available for the accurate chemical estimation of the principal urinary oestrogens (BROWN, 1955; BAULD, 1956) but, although these methods have a high degree of precision and can measure very small quantities, little further information has been gained on any association between urinary oestrogen levels and the behaviour of breast tumours (see pp. 56—57). The principal difficulty is the task of measuring urinary oestrogens throughout many normal menstrual cycles. Variation during the cycle is considerable (BROWN, KLOPPER and LORAINE, 1958) and one isolated estimation would give little useful information. Possibly for this reason, and also because of the low levels usually encountered postmenopausally when cyclical changes are not a problem, no prospective study has yet been undertaken to see whether abnormalities in oestrogen excretion are associated with the development of breast cancer.

In Holland, DE WAARD and his co-workers are measuring oestrogen activity in postmenopausal normal women and relating their results to the subsequent development of breast cancer (BAANDERS-VAN HALEWIJN, 1970). It has been suggested that there are two forms of breast cancer, one occurring principally in premenopausal women and distributed more or less evenly amongst different races, and the other confined mostly to postmenopausal women and having a predominant incidence in Western countries (DE WAARD, BAANDERS-VAN HALEWIJN and HUIZINGA, 1964; DE WAARD, 1970). It is this latter kind which is believed to result from continued postmenopausal oestrogen production ("oestrus"), probably of adrenal origin.

Because urethral cells behave similarly to vaginal cells as a result of oestrogenic stimuli, DE WAARD and his colleagues are using the incidence of squamous and karyopyknotic cells in urinary sediment smears as a measure of hormonal activity. With the help of the local General Practitioners, they are collecting urine specimens from 7,000 normal women between the ages of 55 and 75 living in the Netherlands. In addition to collecting the urine specimens, the blood pressure and weight of each women is recorded because it has been shown that obesity and hypertension are correlated with postmenopausal "oestrus" and also possibly with the incidence of breast cancer (DE WAARD, 1970).

The Dutch study was started in the town of Kampen and has been given the name Kamperfoelie which in English means "honeysuckle" (MULLER, HUISARTS TE KAMPEN and DE WAARD, 1966). It is anticipated that by 1970, 50 cases of breast cancer will occur amongst the women who have taken part, but no results are yet available.

Some investigations have compared the oestrogen excretion of breast cancer patients with that of normal controls, but the results have shown no definite correlations and at times have been conflicting. The principle finding has been that breast cancer patients excrete significantly higher amounts of oestriol. BROWN reported this in 1958, in an investigation of postmenopausal breast cancer patients, and NISSEN-MEYER and SANNER (1963) subsequently described similar findings. MARMORSTON et al. (1965) measured the urinary oestrone, oestradiol and oestriol in 133 pre- and postmenopausal women. These women included breast cancer patients and patients with benign breast disease as well as "sick" and "well" controls. The results showed that the pre- and postmenopausal breast cancer patients excreted a significantly higher proportion of their total oestrogen as oestriol when compared with the "sick" and "well" controls. The premenopausal women with benign breast disease also excreted high levels of oestriol. A dissident finding was reported by LEMON and his colleagues (1966). They measured the proportion of oestriol to oestrone and oestradiol in 26 breast cancer patients and 34 controls. The results show that, irrespective of the menopausal state, the breast cancer patients were excreting less of their total oestrogen as oestriol. Further measurements were made on 53 patients who had either had major ablative procedures or been given hormones to treat the advanced disease. Their oestrogen excretion was similar to that of the control group and LEMON and his colleagues suggested that castration or hormone therapy may "normalise a precancerous metabolic imbalance".

Investigation of the metabolism of administered oestradiol has not shown similar abnormalities to those found in men. HELLMAN et al.(1967) studied the transformation of radioactive oestradiol in 5 healthy postmenopausal women and 11 postmenopausal cancer patients. Within the limits of biological variation, there was no difference between the two groups.

Indirect evidence of an increased oestrogen effect in breast cancer patients has been put forward by ROSE (1967). He had previously shown (ROSE, 1966) that the metabolism of tryptophan could be affected by the administration of oestrogen. In particular, a high dosage of oestrogen resulted in an increased excretion of the three tryptophan metabolites, 3-hydroxykynurenine, xanthurenic acid and 3-hydroxy-anthranilic acid. ROSE administered a tryptophan load to 20 post-mastectomy breast cancer patients, and 15 controls. Subsequent urinary estimations showed that the breast cancer patients were excreting abnormally high quantities of tryptophan metabolites compared with the controls. ROSE suggested that this indicated a high oestrogen effect due either to increased oestrogen secretion or to a defective production of androgens. Measurements were also made on breast cancer patients who had had an oophorectomy. Many of these were found to excrete abnormally low amounts of tryptophan metabolites, presumably as a result of the absence of ovarian oestrogens.

Certain factors such as marriage, parity, breast feeding and early menopause seem to have some influence on the development of breast cancer (see chapter 7). Each of these will be accompanied by an alteration in endogenous oestrogen secretion and may exert their protective effect by this means. On the other hand certain feminising tumours of the ovary secrete abnormally high levels of oestrogen but no data are available that show any association between these tumours and breast cancer. At the present, the relationship between endogenous oestrogen levels and breast cancer incidence is obscure and is further confused by what little data there are available. Although reports both from animal and human investigations would indicate that a high oestrogen effect may be associated with an increased incidence of breast cancer, the correlation is not marked. The findings on disorders of oestriol excretion are interesting and the work needs amplifying. Similarly the inferences from the tryptophan studies are important and further work is needed to clarify the suggestion of an increased oestrogen effect.

The prospective trial in Holland in which the occurrence of postmenopausal "oestrus" as shown by urinary sediment smears is being compared with the subsequent development of breast cancer will be a valuable contribution. Using current methods of measuring urinary oestrogens, a similar trial on oestrogen excretion would involve a vast amount of work but there is sufficient evidence that it would be worthwhile. Further work is needed in oestrogen methodology for such a study to become feasible.

Summary and Conclusions

1. There is suggestive but not conclusive evidence that prolonged administration of oestrogen will cause breast cancer to develop in men.

2. Men with breast cancer metabolise administered oestradiol abnormally.

3. Men with an abnormal endocrine environment have a high incidence of breast cancer.

4. There is no evidence to suggest that oestrogen administration causes breast cancer in women.

5. Women with breast cancer excrete abnormally high amounts of oestriol, but metabolise administered oestradiol normally.

6. There is no evidence to associate high endogenous oestrogen levels with the development of breast cancer in women.

References

ABRAMSON, W., WARSHAWSKY, H.: Cancer of the male breast secondary to oestrogenic administration. J. Urol. **59**, 76 (1948).

ALLABEN, G. R., OWEN, S. E.: Adenocarcinoma of the breast associated with strenuous endocrine therapy. J. Amer. med. Ass. **112**, 1933 (1939).

AUCHINLOSS, H., HAAGENSEN, C. D.: Cancer of the breast possibly induced by oestrogenic substance. J. Amer. med. Ass. **114**, 1517 (1940).

BAANDERS-VAN HALEWIJN, E. A.: Epidemiology of postmenopausal oestrus, studied by means of exfoliative cytology. 18th Year book for cancer research in the Netherlands, 1969, 185.

BAIERL, W.: Zur Frage der Mammacarcinom-Manifestierung nach Cyren B-Behandlung beim Mann. Med. Klin. **48**, 1284 (1953).

BAULD, W. S.: A method for the determination of oestriol and oestradiol-17β in human urine by partition chromatography and colorimetric estimation. Biochem. J. **63**, 488 (1956).

BENSON, W. R.: Carcinoma of the prostate with metastases to breasts and testis; critical review of literature and report of a case. Cancer **10**, 1235 (1957).

— Cancer of the male breast. Brit. med. J. **1965 II**, 171.

BROWN, J. B.: A chemical method for the determination of oestriol, oestrone and oestradiol in the human urine. Biochem. J. **60**, 185 (1955).

— Urinary oestrogen excretion in the study of mammary cancer. In: Endocrine Aspects of Breast Cancer. Ed.: A. R. CURRIE. Edinburgh-London: Livingstone 1958, p. 197.

— KLOPPER, A., LORAINE, J. A.: The urinary examination of oestrogens, pregnanediol and the gonadotrophin during the menstrual cycle. J. Endocr. **17**, 401 (1958).

CAMPBELL, J. H., CUMMINS, S. D.: Metastases simulating mammary cancer in prostatic carcinoma under estrogenic therapy. Cancer **4**, 303 (1951).

CORBETT, D. G., ABRAMS, E. W.: Bilateral carcinoma of the male breast associated with prolonged stilboestrol therapy for carcinoma of the prostate. J. Urol. (Baltimore) **64**, 377 (1950).

DE WAARD, F.: Adrenal oestrogens and the geographical distribution of breast cancer. 18th Year book for cancer research in the Netherlands, 1969, 191.

— BAANDERS-VAN HALEWIJN, E. A., HUIZINGA, J.: The bimodal age distribution of patients with mammary carcinoma. Cancer **17**, 141 (1964).

ENTZ, F. H.: Probable metastatic carcinoma of male breast following stilboestrol therapy. J. Urol. (Baltimore) **59**, 1203 (1948).

FOOTE, F. N., STEWART, F. W.: Comparative studies of cancerous versus non-cancerous breasts. Ann. Surg. **121**, 6, 197 (1945).

GARDINI, G. F.: Gynecomastia con degenerazione cancerigna in prostatico dopo trattamento estrogeno. Oncologia (Basel) **1**, 129 (1948).

GIORGI, E. P., SOMERVILLE, I. F.: Hormone assays in Klinefelter syndrome. J. clin. Endocr. **23**, 197 (1963).

GRAVES, G. Y., HARRIS, H. S.: Carcinoma of the male breast with axillary metastases following stilboestrol therapy. Ann. Surg. **135**, 411 (1952).

GUTHORN, P. J.: Carcinoma of male breast: report of 15 cases. Milit. Surg. **109**, 110 (1951).

HELLER, C. G., NELSON, N. O.: Hypogonadotropic eunuchoidism, its physiology, diagnosis, prognosis and treatment. Proc. Central Soc. Clin. Research. **17**, 74 (1944).

HELLMAN, L., FISHMAN, J., ZUMOFF, B., CASSOUTO, J., GALLAGHER, T. F.: Studies of estradiol transformation in women with breast cancer. J. clin. Endocr. **27**, 1087 (1967).

HERTZ, R.: Relationship between hormone induced tissue growth and neoplasia: review. Cancer Res. 11, 393 (1951).

HOWARD, R. H., GROSJEAN, W. A.: Bilateral mammary carcinoma in the male coincident with prolonged stilboestrol therapy. Surgery 25, 300 (1949).

JACKSON, A. W., MULDAL, S., OCKEY, C. H., O'CONNOR, P. J.: Carcinoma of male breast in association with the Klinefelter syndrome. Brit. med. J. 1965 I, 223.

JAKOBSEN, A. H. J.: Bilateral mammary carcinoma in the male following stilboestrol therapy. Acta path. microbiol. scand. 31, 60 (1952).

LACCASSAGNE, A.: Apparition de cancer de la mamelle chez la souris male, soumis a des injections de folliculine. Compt. Rend. Acad. Sci. 195, 630 (1932).

LEMON, H. E., WOTIZ, H. H., PARSONS, L., MOZDEN, P. H.: Reduced estriol excretion in patients with breast cancer prior to endocrine therapy. J. Amer. med. Ass. 196, 1128 (1966).

LIEBEGOTT, G.: Mammacarcinom beim Mann nach Follikelhormonbehandlung. Klin. Wschr. 26, 599 (1948).

LILIENFELD, A. M.: The epidemiology of breast cancer. Cancer Res. 23, 1503 (1963).

MARMORSTON, J., CROWLEY, L. G., MYERS, S. M., STERN, E., HOPKINS, C. E.: Urinary excretion of estrone, estradiol and estriol by patients with breast cancer and benign breast disease. Amer. J. Obstet. Gynec. 92, 460 (1965).

McCLURE, J. A.: Male breast carcinoma and estrogen therapy. J. Amer. med. Ass. 146, 1608 (1951).

— HIGGINS, C. C.: Bilateral carcinoma of male breast after estrogen therapy. J. Amer. med. Ass. 146, 7 (1951).

MULLER, H. K., HUISARTS TE KAMPEN, DE WAARD, F.: Het project "Kamperfoelie". Huisarts en Wetenschap 9, 307 (1966).

NISSEN-MEYER, R., SANNER, T.: The excretion of oestrone, pregnanediol and pregnanetriol in breast cancer patients. II. Effect of ovariectomy, ovarian irradiation and corticosteroids. Acta endocr. 44, 334 (1963).

PARSONS, W. H., McCALL, E. F.: The role of oestrogenic substances in the production of malignant mammary lesions. Surgery 9, 780 (1941).

ROSE, D. P.: The influence of oestrogens on tryptophan metabolism in man. Clin. Sci. 31, 265 (1966).

— Tryptophan metabolism in carcinoma of the breast. Lancet 1967 I, 239.

SHIMKIN, M. B., WYMAN, R. S.: Mammary tumours in male mice implanted with estrogen-cholestrol pellets. J. nat. Cancer Inst. 7, 71 (1946).

SYMMERS, W. ST. C.: Carcinoma of the breast in trans-sexual individuals after surgical and hormonal interference with the primary and secondary sex characteristics. Brit. med. J. 1968 I, 83.

TREVES, N., HOLLEB, A. I.: Cancer of male breast: report of 146 cases. Cancer 8, 1239 (1955).

WAGGONER, C. M.: Carcinoma of the premenopausal breast. Endocrine influence suggested clinically in 31 cases. Ann. Surg. 127, 1256 (1948).

WILSON, R. H.: The roles of estrogen and progesterone in breast and genital cancer. J. Amer. med. Ass. 182, 327 (1962).

ZUMMOFF, B., FISHMAN, J., CASSOUTO, J., HELLMAN, L., GALLAGHER, T. F.: Estradiol transformation in men with breast cancer. J. clin. Endocr. 26, 960 (1966).

Chapter 9

Androgens and Corticosteroids

BULBROOK (1965) in his review on hormone assays in human breast cancer writes "... an essential feature in any study of the endocrine aspects of breast cancer is a measure of the hormone responsiveness of the tumour. Without this information, the normal hormonal environment found in so many patients, may obscure the fact that an abnormal environment may be found in the rest." This statement has particular application in studies carried out on the part played by androgens and corticosteroids in the development of breast cancer. It was not until patients with breast cancer were considered as two populations, with either hormone responsive or hormone unresponsive tumours, that consistent abnormalities in androgen excretion were noted. The demonstration of these abnormalities was delayed because for a long time most workers in this field were pre-occupied with measuring oestrogen excretion, an approach which theoretically seemed logical but which in practice, provided little useful information.

Interest turned to the investigation of endogenous androgens and in 1960 BULBROOK, GREENWOOD and HAYWARD showed that the preoperative urinary levels of the 11-deoxy-17-oxosteroids and the 17-OHCS, combined as a discriminant function, varied according to the subsequent response of the patient to adrenalectomy or hypophysectomy (see page 60).

Subsequently, BULBROOK and his colleagues (1962 a) reported (see page 79) that the distribution of the discriminant was similar in patients with early and advanced breast cancer. In either case, they found that about one third of the patients had positive discriminants and two thirds had negative discriminants. In the advanced disease, the patients with negative discriminants did badly after subsequent ablation and in the early disease, the patients with negative discriminants had a poor prognosis following mastectomy (BULBROOK et al., 1964) (see pages 80—81). The scattergrams illustrated in Fig. 16 a and b show that there was no correlation between the discriminant and age in the patients with breast cancer. The distribution of positives and negatives seemed random, irrespective of whether the patients was young or old.

The discriminant function was calculated to obtain the best possible prediction of success or failure in patients awaiting endocrine ablation. Although the value of the discriminant depended on the preoperative levels of aetiocholanolone and the 17-OHCS, there was little evidence of its physiological meaning. Also there was no information on the distribution of positive and negative discriminants in the normal population.

In 1962 b, BULBROOK et al. reported an investigation comparing the urinary steroid excretion of normal women with that of women with advanced breast cancer.

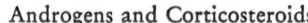

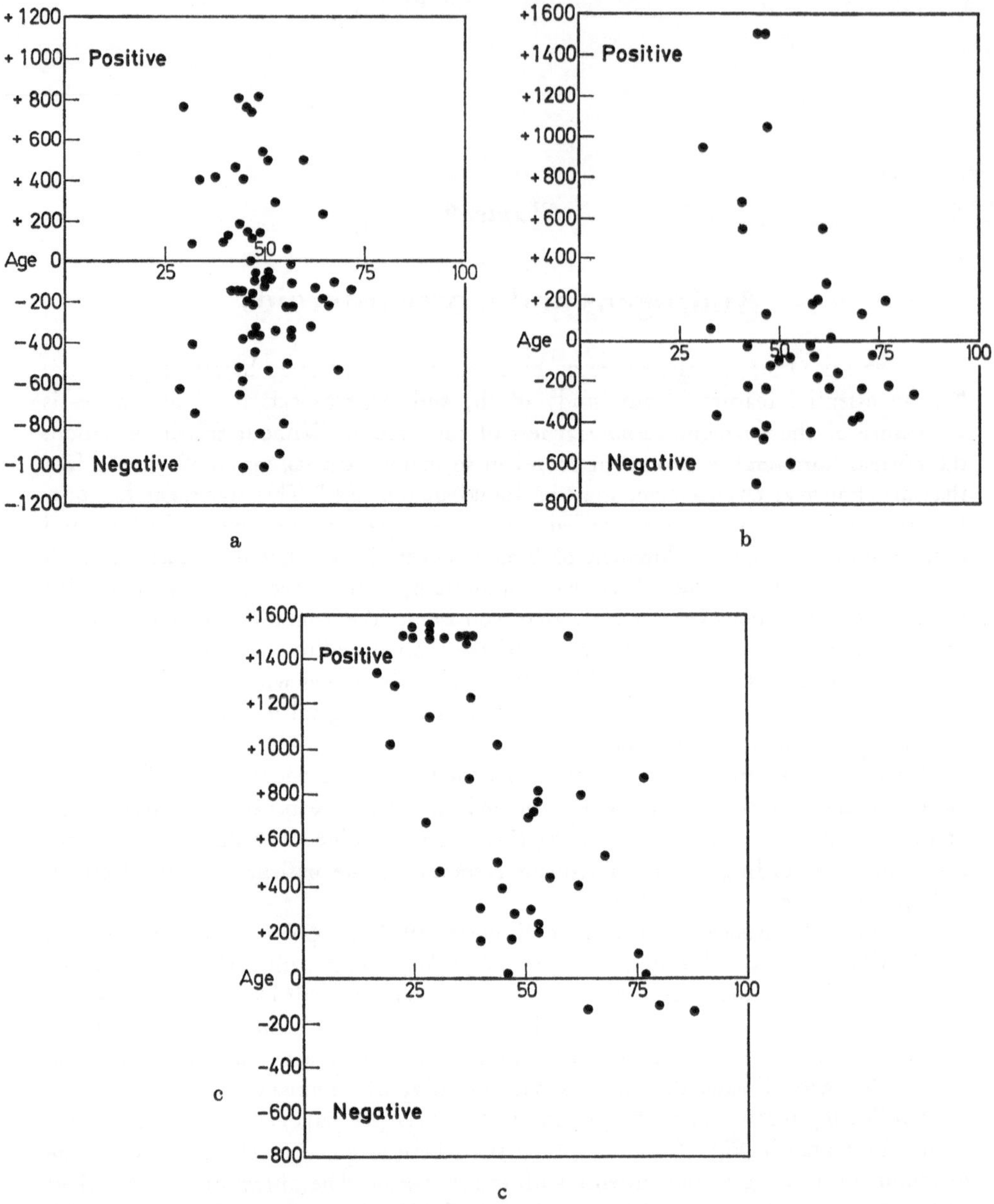

Fig. 16. The distribution of the discriminant in patients with (a) advanced breast cancer and, (b) early breast cancer; (c) shows the distribution in normal women

Seventy women with the advanced disease were studied and their hormone excretion was measured on three or five day samples collected immediately before endocrine ablation. In the control series, the same hormones were measured in single 24-hour specimens, obtained from normal women between the ages of seventeen and eighty-eight; these women were not hospitalized. Estimations of the urinary 11-deoxy-

17-oxosteroids and the 17-OHCS in the normal women showed that the hormone levels were indistinguishable from those in the women with advanced breast cancer who subsequently responded to adrenalectomy or hypophysectomy. Calculation of the discriminant in the normal women showed that the results were positive in all cases, except in those aged sixty-five or over. Negative discriminants did not occur in the normal population aged under sixty-five.

The distribution of the discriminants in these groups—normal women, women with early breast cancer and women with advanced breast cancer—is compared in Fig. 16 a, b and c. This shows another feature of the discriminant in the normal women which was not shown in either the early or advanced cancer groups. Not only were there no negative discriminants in the normals aged under sixty-five, but also the value of the discriminant in the normals decreased with age. This regression with age was not found in either of the cancer groups, except in the advanced patients who responded to endocrine ablation (BULBROOK et al., 1962 a, b).

To summarise, positive discriminants are derived from normal hormone levels. They were found in the normal population aged under sixty-five, in early breast cancer patients who had a good prognosis following mastectomy and in advanced breast cancer patients who did well after adrenalectomy or hypophysectomy. Negative discriminants are derived from abnormal hormone levels, and they were not found in the normal population except in the elderly. Some two thirds of the early breast cancer patients had negative discriminants and these patients tended to recur soon after mastectomy. The patients with advanced disease who had negative discriminants failed to respond to adrenalectomy or hypophysectomy. In addition, there was no correlation between the discriminant and age in patients with breast cancer other than those who responded to ablation, whereas there was a positive regression with age in normal women.

The finding of negative discriminants—indicating an abnormal steroid excretion—in some women with early breast cancer posed the important question of how the abnormalities developed. The changes in steroid excretion probably resulted from alterations in hormone secretion or metabolism, but their relationship to the development of the tumour was unknown. On the one hand, the abnormalities may have developed at the same time as, and as a result of, the clinical appearance of the disease, yet it seemed unlikely that a small amount of tumour tissue could have such a profound effect on endocrine excretion. Alternatively, the hormone abnormalities could have developed long before the clinical appearance of the disease and possibly, even before the formation of the tumour. In other words, those patients with negative discriminants may have exhibited abnormalities in androgen and corticoid excretion for many years, possibly from puberty or soon after. If this was so, the hormone abnormalities might be associated with the factors involved in transforming normal breast cells into malignant ones. Moreover, by carrying out the relevant hormone assays, it might be possible to identify such patients before the clinical appearance of the disease.

The test of the thesis was to measure the hormone excretion of a large number of women, and to see if those who developed breast cancer had an abnormal steroid excretion. Such an experiment has been carried out during the past few years on the island of Guernsey and the preliminary results have been reported (BULBROOK and HAYWARD, 1967).

The Guernsey Trial

The purpose of this trial was to measure the hormone excretion in a large number of ostensibly normal women and to see whether those who subsequently developed breast cancer had an abnormal steroid excretion before diagnosis. It was estimated that about 5,000 women, aged from thirty-five to fifty-five, would be needed. Women over fifty-five were excluded because the hormone measurements tend to be unreliable in older women, and women under thirty-five were excluded because they would have only a slight chance of developing breast cancer during the period of the present investigation. In fact, the lower age limit was reduced from thirty-five to thirty later in the study.

In Great Britain, breast cancer occurs at an approximate rate of one case per 800 women per year. It was estimated that if urines were collected from a thousand women every year, by the end of five years some 5,000 women would have been studied and seventeen cases of breast cancer would have occurred amongst them; a number which would be sufficient for at least a preliminary analysis to be made.

There was much debate on the most suitable geographical site for conducting such an experiment. The most obvious and most convenient place would have been London: the analyses were to be carried out at the Imperial Cancer Research Fund Laboratories which are situated there and it should not have been difficult to persuade 5,000 London women to take part. But there were also considerable problems in choosing such a large city. Five per cent of the population of London move every year so that at the end of five years, nearly 25 per cent of the women would have left the area, making follow-up more difficult. Also, reliance would have to be placed on the General Practitioners and hospitals to report when a case of breast cancer had occurred in those women who had given urine samples; but there are too many doctors and hospitals in the London area to ensure 100 per cent notification. A stable community was needed covering a small area and having only a few doctors and hospitals to which women could report if they had breast disease. An island community seemed ideal and for convenience of size and access, it was decided to attempt the study on Guernsey in the Channel Islands. Guernsey is one of a group of small islands lying off the coast of Normandy; it is a British Crown Dependency and easily reached by air and boat services from England. In 1961, the population of Guernsey (including the neighbouring islands of Alderney and Sark) was just over 48,000. The inhabitants are either of British or French stock and both languages are still spoken. Although English is the principal language, many of the people—particularly in the country areas—still speak French patois. The incidence of breast cancer in the Island is similar to that in the United Kingdom. There is no National Health Service on Guernsey and at that time the medical service was provided by twenty-three doctors and one hospital. It was estimated that there were about 8,000 women available within the required age groups.

In October 1961, the proposed scheme was described to a meeting of the local doctors who agreed to co-operate by supplying information on those patients who took part; in particular they were asked to notify the organisers of the study should any of their patients develop breast cancer. Requests for volunteers were made through the press (there were two local daily newspapers), the island television service and particularly through the local women's organisations.

A nurse was employed full-time in Guernsey to collect the specimens. She delivered a two litre plastic bottle to the houses of the women who had volunteered to take part. Instructions were given for carrying out a 24-hour save which was usually completed over a week-end. The containers were collected on the following day. The urine was immediately deep frozen and stored to await transport to the mainland. Each volunteer was also asked to complete a questionnaire, detailing her age, height, weight, menstrual history, etc.; these data were later transferred to a punch-card.

Urines were collected at a rate of twenty five per week; following storage at $-20°$ C, they were transported by air to London in batches of about fifty. They arrived at the London laboratories on the same day and still frozen. The estimations of the urinary 17-OHCS were carried out soon after the urines arrived but the 11-deoxy-17-oxosteroids were not measured. Instead, an extract of the urine was obtained and stored in a cold room at $-20°$ C. The principal reason for not measuring the 11-deoxy-17-oxosteroids immediately was that at the beginning of the study the methods of measurement were very laborious, and facilities were not available for carrying out the estimations on such a large number of specimens. More recently, the use of gas chromatography has greatly simplified the assays and has enabled the estimations to be carried out on all the specimens soon after they are received.

Every month each doctor on Guernsey received a list of the names of his patients who had taken part in the experiment. This enabled him to mark their notes so that if they developed any illness he would be reminded that they had taken part in the scheme. The doctors were asked to report the occurrence of any form of cancer, particularly breast cancer; also information was requested on the development of coronary artery disease and any form of endocrine dyscrasia. To ensure that no cases were missed, the Guernsey Hospital records were searched once a year.

When a case of breast cancer was reported, a section of the histological specimen was obtained, both to confirm the diagnosis and to grade the tumour. Whenever possible, a further 24 hour urine specimen was collected from the patients before mastectomy and again ten days after mastectomy. Subsequently urine specimens were collected every six months. Using the punch cards the cancer patient was then matched against ten or twelve controls. In addition, another serial number was chosen at random to act as a pseudo-cancer case. To obviate bias, the matching was carried out "blind" so that it was not known which was the cancer case and which was the pseudo-cancer case. The serial numbers were matched for age, menstrual status, weight, height, parity and number of children, in that order. These numbers—that is the numbers of the cancer cases and their controls and the numbers of the pseudo-cancer cases and their controls—were sent to the laboratory but without identification. The estimations were then completed on the stored urine extracts corresponding to these numbers, and only when the assays were completed was the code broken and the numbers of the cancer cases and the pseudo-cancer cases made known.

4,850 urines were collected during the first five and a half years of the study and nineteen cases of breast cancer were reported during this time. Two of the breast cancer cases had to be discarded; one because of myxoedema (thyroid dysfunction markedly affects the excretion of androgen metabolites and the 17-OHCS—and hence the discriminant—see GALLAGHER et al., 1960; SNEDDON, STEEL and

STRONG, 1968) and the other because the urinary creatinine levels were unsatisfactory. This left seventeen cases for analysis. All the urines had been collected before the breast cancer had become clinically manifest and there was a mean interval of thirty one months between the collection and the diagnosis of cancer. The shortest interval was three months and the longest, sixty-one months.

In the analysis of the results, it was decided not to rely on the concept of the discriminant function. Essentially, two measurements had been made— the levels of the 17-OHCS and of aetiocholanolone—and for each cancer case and set of controls, a mean level could be calculated for each of these hormones.

It was decided to see if the hormone levels of the cancer cases deviated further from the mean levels of their groups than did the hormone levels of the controls. The variance differed widely between the sets of controls. To compensate for this, for each set of controls the differences from the mean were divided by the standard deviation. The result of this calculation was termed the "weighted deviation" and the greater the value for the weighted deviation, the more aberrant were the values of the 17-OHCS or the aetiocholanolone from the group mean.

The combined individual weighted distances for the 17-OHCS and aetiocholanolone were termed the "weighted square distances". For example, Fig. 17 illustrates the differences from the mean for cancer patient No. 2 and her five controls. Table 22 shows the calculation of the weighted deviations and the weighted square distances in this case.

Table 22. *Method of calculating the weighted square distance for case 2.* (BULBROOK and HAYWARD, 1967)

Volunteer	17-OHCS (mg/24 hrs.) (x)	Aetio-cholanolone (mg/24 hrs.) (y)	Weighted deviations 17-OHCS $d_x = (x - \bar{x})/s_x$	Weighted deviations aetio-cholanolone $d_y = (y - \bar{y})/s_y$	Weighted square distance $d^2 = d_x^2 + d_y^2$
Control	8.20	1.860	+0.37	+1.223	1.64
Control	9.50	1.360	+0.88	+0.141	0.80
Control	5.70	1.678	−0.60	+0.829	1.05
Control	10.60	1.290	+1.31	−0.011	1.72
Control	5.20	1.006	−0.80	−0.625	1.02
Cancer case	4.23	0.578	−1.17	−1.550	3.78

Mean $\bar{x} = 7.24$; $\bar{y} = 1.295$
Standard deviation: $s_x = 2.57$; $s_y = 0.462$

The weighted deviations were plotted as co-ordinates (Fig. 18), and the more a value lay on the periphery of this plot, the more it deviated from the mean. In Fig. 18, a line has been drawn joining the majority of the cancer cases, and shows that they tend to lie on the periphery; this peripheral tendency was statistically significant. This meant that, in the Guernsey trial, most of the seventeen women who developed breast cancer had had an abnormality of urinary hormone excretion before the disease had become clinically apparent. This abnormality was in the excretion of the 17-OHCS and aetiocholanolone and was multidirectional (although

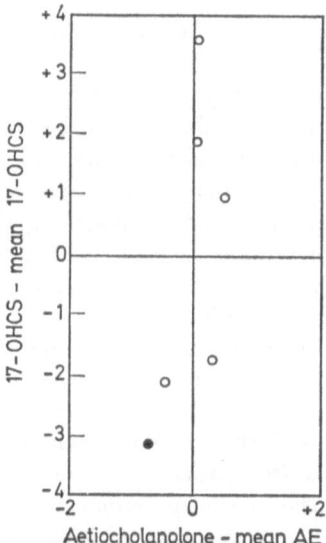

Fig. 17. The 17-OHCS and aetiocholanolone values expressed as deviations from the mean in cancer case No. 2 (mean 17-OHCS, 7.24 mg per 24 hours; mean aetiocholanolone, 1.30 mg per 24 hours) (replotted from data in BULBROOK and HAYWARD, 1967)

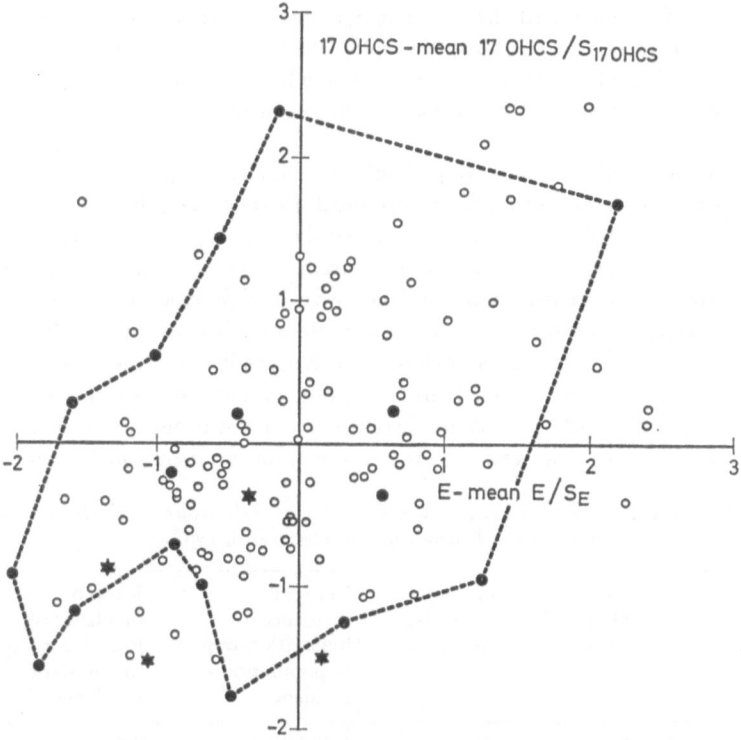

Fig. 18. The weighted deviations of the individual 17-OHCS and aetiocholanolone values plotted as co-ordinates. To indicate the peripheral tendency, the plots for the majority of the cancer cases have been jointed by a dotted line. The large black circles represent the cancer cases, the small open circles represent the controls and the asteriks represent the four subsequent cancer cases. (Replotted from data in BULBROOK, HAYWARD and ALLEN, 1969)

the principal abnormality seemed to be subnormal excretion of aetiocholanolone). Because the women had not been examined when their urine had been collected, it was not precisely known whether this abnormality had preceeded the onset of the disease. Indeed, it was likely that in many of the cases, especially those with a short interval between the urine collection and the diagnosis, the disease must have been present but not giving rise to symptoms. Nevertheless, it was felt that the results lent some credence to the hypothesis that abnormalities in steroid production were associated with the aetiology of breast cancer.

In a subsequent report, BULBROOK, HAYWARD and ALLEN (1969) described a further four cases of breast cancer that had occurred in the Guernsey trial. Like the original seventeen cases, three of these four women excreted in their urine amounts of aetiocholanolone and the 17-OHCS which significantly differed from those found in their controls (see patients indicated by an asterisk in Fig. 18). BULBROOK et al. (1969) also measured these steroids in the urine of twelve unaffected sisters of the Guernsey patients. When compared with controls, many of these sisters were also excreting abnormal amounts of aetiocholanolone and the 17-OHCS. Fig. 19 shows that the pattern of excretion in the sisters is similar to that demonstrated in the cancer cases. Although all these sisters were ostensibly normal when their urine was collected, those marked with arrows in Fig. 19 have since developed breast cancer. Sisters of women with breast cancer have 2—3 time the normal chance of developing the disease (see page 99). In view of the abnormalities already demonstrated in the urine of many of those women who subsequently developed breast cancer, the finding of similar abnormalities in the urine of their sisters is not unexpected.

The descriptions of the Guernsey Trial were interim reports and it would be unwise to read too much into the results until further cases have been analysed. Nevertheless, two possibilities for further study are suggested. Firstly, there is the possibility of using urinary steroid measurements as a method of screening the general population to identify women who have a high risk of developing breast cancer. To do this, it would be necessary to choose a critical distance from the group mean in Fig. 18 and if a woman's hormone levels were beyond this critical distance, she would be considered to be in a high risk group. BULBROOK and HAYWARD (1967) calculated the possible risk at various distances from the group mean and these are given in Table 23. It can be seen that if a proportion is taken which would include

Table 23. *The incidence of breast cancer in high and low risk groups, calculated for various percentiles.* (BULBROOK and HAYWARD, 1967)

Critical value (percentile)	% of population in: High-risk group	Low-risk group	Ratio of incidence of high-risk group to population incidence	Ratio of incidence of low-risk group to population incidence
50th	50	50	1.65	0.35
60th	40	60	1.62	0.59
70th	30	70	1.96	0.42
80th	20	80	2.35	0.67
90th	10	90	1.77	0.20

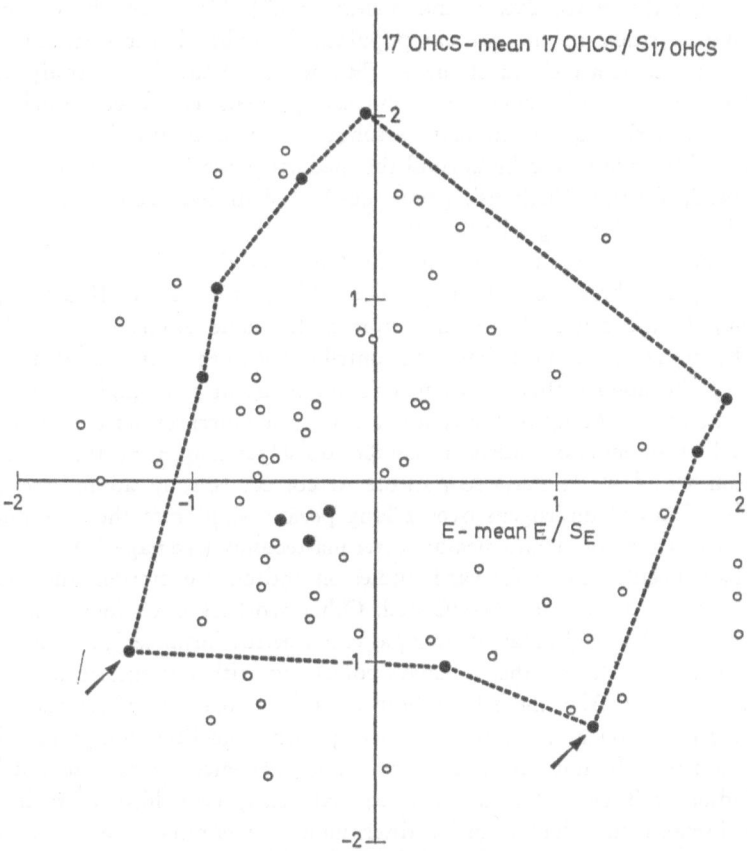

Fig. 19. The weighted deviations of the individual 17-OHCS and aetiocholanolone values for the sisters of the Guernsey cancer cases plotted as co-ordinates. To indicate the peripheral tendency, the plots for the majority of the sisters have been joined by a line. The large black circles represent the sisters, and the small open circles represent the controls. The two sisters whose plots have been arrowed have since developed breast cancer. (Replotted from data in BULBROOK, HAYWARD and ALLEN, 1969)

20 per cent of the population, the incidence of breast cancer in this group might be 2.35 times higher than that found in the total population.

The importance of this high risk group lies in the application that might then be made of more precise techniques for detecting cancer in its very early stages. Combined mammography and clinical examination appears to be a practical method for the early detection of breast cancer—tumours which are impalpable clinically sometimes can be identified by mammography. In New York, a study is being carried out in which a group of women is undergoing annual mammography and clinical examination in an attempt to detect very early breast cancers. The incidence is being compared with that of women in a control group who have no routine examinations but report to their doctor in the usual way if they discover a lump in the breast. In the first year of examination, approximately twice as many cancer cases were detected in the study group than in the control group and these cancers were at an earlier stage (SHAPIRO, STRAX and VENET, 1967). However, the economics of applying such a study to the general population would almost certainly make it impractical for use as a method of survey (HAYWARD, 1966). In the study described by SHAPIRO and his colleagues, only thirteen patients could be examined in a 3^1/$_4$ hour session; the equipment and personnel required to provide such a service on a nation-wide scale would be beyond the medical potential of most countries. On the other hand, if a small high-risk group could be identified, regular mammography and clinical examination might be feasible.

The second possibility arising from the Guernsey Trial is that some form of prophylaxis against breast cancer may be possible in the future. If many patients who develop breast cancer have an abnormal hormone environment and if this abnormal hormone environment has been contributory to the initiation of the disease, correction of the abnormality in women found to be at risk might in those cases prevent breast cancer. Many of the cancer cases in the Guernsey series were excreting abnormally low amounts of androgen metabolites which may mean that their androgen secretion was low. It may be possible to correct this by administering small non-virilising doses of androgens over a long period, similar to the way androgens are being tried as a prophylactic measure after mastectomy (see page 79).

There have been no other forward studies on androgen excretion, and the results of the Guernsey trial remain unconfirmed. Other workers have found similar hormone changes in advanced breast cancer patients (see for instance JURET et al., 1964; KUMAOKA et al., 1968), and these changes correlated with response to ablative procedures (see page 65). Also there have been some investigations where the androgen and corticoid excretion of early breast cancer patients has been compared with that of normal controls. In most instances significant differences were observed but the original finding of BULBROOK et al. (1962 a) that nearly two thirds of their patients with early breast cancer had negative discriminants was almost certainly an overestimate and has not been confirmed by subsequent investigation. For instance, MILLER and DURANT (1968), using a ratio of the total 11-deoxy-17-oxosteroids to the 17-OHCS (a function which closely mimics the value of the discriminant—see page 65) found abnormally low values in only 14 per cent of their premenopausal early breast cancer patients.

In two instances, no differences could be demonstrated between the steroid excretion of breast cancer patients and controls. SCHWEPPE, JUNGMAN and LEWIN (1967) measured the total urinary 17-oxosteroids in normal postmenopausal women, postmastectomy patients without recurrence and patients with metastatic breast cancer. In each case the steroid excretion was measured under basal conditions, following corticotrophic stimulation and following dexamethasone suppression. They found that the cancer patients excreted slightly higher amounts of 17-oxosteroids than the normal group in all conditions under test. They did not think these differences were significant because all the measurements were within an expected normal range. In fact, only 16 patients were studied—six normals, five early cancers and five metastatic cancers—and, in addition, no attempt was made to group the cancer patients according to the hormone responsiveness of their tumours. WADE et al. (1969) measured the discriminant in 32 normal women, 33 women who were in hospital for operations on conditions other than breast cancer and 26 women who were admitted for mastectomy. They observed that the values for the breast patients did not differ significantly at any age from those of the controls, and considered that the discriminant was not significantly affected in breast cancer.

Other investigations have tended to confirm the findings of BULBROOK and his colleagues (1962 a, b). SNEDDON et al. (1968) found that the discriminant was significantly lower in 20 early breast cancer patients than in the same number of controls. In their patients, the low value of the discriminant was the result of a low excretion of aetiocholanolone; the 17-OHCS excretion was normal. BACIGALUPO and LINGK (1968) measured the urinary excretion of the neutral 17-oxosteroids, androsterone and aetiocholanolone in 26 healthy women, 27 patients with early breast cancer and 37 patients with advanced breast cancer. All but two of the women were postmenopausal. Irrespective of the stage of the cancer, the women with breast cancer excreted significantly lower amounts of the neutral 17-oxosteroids than the normal women. Although there was little difference in the excretion of aetiocholanolone between the three groups, the breast cancer patients excreted significantly less androsterone than the normal women. In a similar experiment, GUTIERREZ and WILLIAMS (1967) measured the excretion of seven individual oxosteroids (androsterone, aetiocholanolone and dehydroepiandrosterone—the 11-deoxy-17-oxosteroids and products of androgen metabolism—and 11-hydroxyandrosterone, 11-hydroxyaetiocholanolone, 11-ketoandrosterone and 11-ketoaetiocholanolone—the 11-oxy-17-oxosteroids and products of cortisol metabolism) in eight premenopausal women after mastectomy and ten matched normal controls. They observed that the cancer patients excreted significantly less aetiocholanolone, 11-hydroxyaetiocholanolone, 11-keto-aetiocholanolone and total 17-oxosteroids than the healthy controls. They concluded that distinctive patterns of oxosteroid excretion were definitely associated with breast cancer, and that in susceptible individuals proneness to the disease could probably be detected beforehand.

MARMORSTON et al. (1967) measured the fractionated 11-deoxy-17-oxosteroids in 114 women; fifty-six of these women were premenopausal and fifty-eight postmenopausal. The premenopausal women were divided into four groups (breast cancer, benign breast disease, sick controls and well controls). The levels of aetiocholanolone and androsterone excreted by the premenopausal breast cancer patients were significantly lower than the levels excreted by the other premenopausal groups and were not significantly different from the levels of postmenopausal cancer patients. MARMORSTON and her associates were not able to explain these findings by the debility of the patients and considered that their results confirmed those of BULBROOK et al. (1962).

Plasma Studies

Whilst the urinary excretion of androgens and corticosteroids has been studied fairly extensively, far less work has been done on the measurement of these hormones in blood. Although methods for the estimation of many plasma steroids have been available for some time, little progress has been made in applying these assays to the study of breast cancer. This is unfortunate because future developments in the use of hormone assays in breast cancer may rely on the more sophisticated measurements that can be done on samples of plasma or blood. The urine studies have revealed many fruitful lines of research but for many reasons urine is an unsatisfactory medium with which to work. There are certain inherent practical difficulties in obtaining specimens of urine which have to be collected over a long period of time. This is particularly so in women who are not in hospital when there is always some uncertainty whether the urine specimen is complete. Frequently, smaller specimens have to be used than would be considered ideal. Also, urinary steroid levels are subject to variations which are often due to factors entirely beyond the control of the observer and sometimes unknown to him. Compounds are assayed which represent the end of a long metabolic chain and consequently the measurements are a very indirect guide to the conditions *in vivo*. On the other hand, blood samples can be obtained under controlled conditions. The time of sampling, the quantity of blood taken and its treatment immediately after collection can be precise. Specimens can be taken quickly and the variables are reduced to a minimum.

Of most value in the investigation of the hormonal background in breast cancer would be information on the rates of secretion of the different hormones believed to be involved in the aetiology and development of the disease. Measurement of the secretion rates of androgens and androgen metabolites have been attempted but the results have largely been invalidated by methodological difficulties. The methods so far used have depended on the administration of a radio-active compound and the measurement of it's dilution by the naturally occurring compound. This should give an indication of the contribution of the natural compound to the total amount assayed, and hence of its secretion rate. One difficulty in this type of estimation is that there may be more than one secretory product of a compound. Attempts have been made to compensate for this by administering tracer doses of two compounds —representing two secretory products—simultaneously.

To date, attempts to measure secretion rates have contributed little to our understanding of the mechanisms which may be responsible for an abnormal hormone excretion in women with breast cancer. BULBROOK et al. (1963) measured the secretion rates of dehydroepiandrosterone (which is a precursor of both androsterone and aetiocholanolone) and cortisol in patients with the advanced disease. Although the methods used for measuring the secretion rate of dehydroepiandrosterone did not take into account other secretory products, it was inferred that the abnormalities that had previously been noted in androgen excretion (BULBROOK et al., 1962 b), could be accounted for by a diminished secretion of dehydroepiandrosterone. They also reported that cortisol secretion rates in their cancer and control groups were similar.

Relatively more work has been done on measuring plasma steroid levels than on estimating secretion rates. For instance, DESHPANDE, HAYWARD and BULBROOK (1965) estimated the levels of the 17-OHCS in urine and plasma of normal women, patients with early breast cancer and patients with advanced breast cancer. They showed that the mean 17-OHCS levels in plasma were normal in patients with early breast cancer but raised in those with the advanced disease; in each case the variance was significantly greater than in normal women. But, when plasma and urinary estimations of the 17-OHCS were compared in the same advanced breast cancer patients, no correlation could be found. The estimations of the urinary 17-OHCS in some of the patients had been abnormally high but this was not associated with a corresponding rise in the plasma titres. Similar discrepancies in urinary and plasma levels of the 17-OHCS in advanced breast cancer patients have been described elsewhere (see for instance BECK et al., 1965). DESHPANDE et al. (1965) comment that the situation is similar to that found in pregnant or oestrogen treated women where a high plasma 17-OHCS concentration is associated with a high level of transcortin but not with an increase in the urinary 17-OHCS.

BELL et al. (1967) measured the transcortin levels in normal women, patients with benign breast disease and patients with early or advanced breast cancer. They found a significantly greater variation in the transcortin levels of cancer patients, compared with normal women; this resulted from the very low levels of cortisol binding found in some of the cancer patients. They comment that this is probably the reason for the failure of DESHPANDE et al. (1965) to find a correlation between the urinary and plasma 17-OHCS values in advanced breast cancer patients.

BELL et al. (1967) further suggest that the obesity, diabetes and impaired glucose tolerance which are reported to be common in breast cancer patients (see for instance DE WAARD et al., 1964) may stem from an excessive adrenocortical stimulus and may precede the clinical appearance of the disease. In normal women, a low cortisol binding capacity is also associated with diminished carbohydrate tolerance and obesity (DE MOOR, HENDRIKS and STEENO, 1965). BELL and her colleagues suggest that the abnormal transcortin levels may also precede the appearance of breast cancer and in turn be responsible for the observed abnormalities in carbohydrate metabolism and obesity found in patients with this disease.

The available information on the plasma levels of the 17-oxosteroids is even less precise. According to DESHPANDE and BULBROOK (1964) the main representatives of the 17-oxosteroids in the plasma are dehydroepiandrosterone sulphate and androsterone sulphate. DESHPANDE et al. (1965) measured the plasma 17-oxosteroid levels in normal women and patients with early and advanced breast cancer. They found that the levels of the cancer patients did not differ significantly from the normals, although the variance was increased. They compared the plasma with the urinary 17-oxosteroid levels in patients with advanced breast cancer and found a significant correlation. Other workers found differences in the plasma 17-oxosteroid levels between normal women and patients with breast cancer. BENARD et al. (1962) found the levels significantly raised in postmenopausal women with breast cancer when compared with controls; premenopausal women with breast cancer had normal levels.

Measurements have also been made of free testosterone levels in the plasma of women with breast cancer. WANG, HAYWARD and BULBROOK (1966) estimated the plasma testosterone in fourteen women with benign breast disease, twenty-four women with early breast cancer and nineteen normal women. There was no correlation between the plasma testosterone levels and age in any of these groups of patients nor did the mean levels differ between the groups. The plasma testosterone concentration was also compared with the levels of androsterone and aetiocholanolone in the urine but no correlation could be detected.

WANG and his colleagues concluded that the abnormal excretion of urinary metabolites in patients with breast cancer did not reflect deficient levels of plasma testosterone. They further suggested that simultaneous measurements of androstenedione and testosterone in the plasma, coupled with a further investigation into the secretion rates of dehydroepiandrosterone and dehydroepiandrosterone sulphate, would be needed before an accurate assessment of the androgenic status of these patients could be made.

Summary and Conclusions

1. Many women with breast cancer excrete abnormal amounts of the 17-OHCS and 11-deoxy-17-oxosteroids.

2. In these patients the tumour recurs rapidly after mastectomy and in the late disease it fails to respond to ablative procedures.

3. In normal women, there is a positive correlation between age and the urinary levels of the 17-OHCS and 11-deoxy-17-oxosteroids. In breast cancer patients, there is no such correlation except in those who respond to ablative procedures.

4. A prospective trial has been carried out to investigate the hormone excretion of women who subsequently develop breast cancer.

5. Preliminary results have shown that many of these women are excreting abnormal amounts of the 17-OHCS and aetiocholanolone up to 6 years before the disease presents clinically.

6. Similar abnormalities have been found in the urine of sisters of women with breast cancer.

7. These findings may enable a high risk group to be identified in the general population.

8. In breast cancer patients, no correlation has been found between the levels of the 17-OHCS in urine and plasma. This may be due to abnormalities in the levels of transcortin.

9. Findings on plasma 17-oxosteroid levels in breast cancer patients and controls have been conflicting.

References

BACIGALUPO, VON G., LINGK, H.: Die Urinausscheidung von neutralen 17-Ketosteroiden, Androsteron und Ätiocholanolon bei gesunden Frauen und Frauen mit frühem und vorgeschrittenem Brustkrebs. Arch. Geschwulstforsch. 32, 95 (1968).

BECK, J. C., BLAIR, A. J., GRIFFITHS, M. M., ROSENFELD, M. W., McGARRY, E. E.: In search of hormonal factors as an aid in predicting the outcome of breast carcinoma. In: Proceedings of the Sixth Canadian Cancer Conference. Ed.: R. W. BEGG. Oxford: Pergamon Press 1966, p. 3.

BELL, E., BULBROOK, R. D., DESHPANDE, N.: Transcortin in the plasma of patients with breast cancer. Lancet 1967 II, 395.

BÉNARD, H., BOURDIN, J. S., SARACINO, R. T., SEEMAN, A.: Study of the plasma 17-ketosteroids in 51 cases of breast cancer. Ann. endocr. (Paris) 23, 525 (1962).

BULBROOK, R. D.: Hormone assays in human breast cancer. Vitam. and Horm. 23, 329 (1965).

— GREENWOOD, F. C., HAYWARD, J. L.: Selection of breast-cancer patients for adrenalectomy or hypophysectomy by determination of urinary 17-hydroxycorticosteroids and aetiocholanolone. Lancet 1960 I, 1154.

— HAYWARD, J. L.: Abnormal urinary steroid excretion and subsequent breast cancer. Lancet 1967 I, 519.

— — ALLEN, D. S.: Further observations on steroid excretion and subsequent breast cancer in a prospective study. 18th Year book for cancer research in the Netherlands, 1969, p. 163.

— — SALOKONGAS, R. A. A.: The secretion rates of dehydroepiandrosterone and cortisol in patients with advanced breast cancer. J. Endocr. 26, i—ii (1963).

— — SPICER, C. C., THOMAS, B. S.: Abnormal excretion of urinary steroids by women with early breast cancer. Lancet 1962 II a, 1238.

— — — — A comparison between the urinary steroid excretion of normal women and women with advanced breast cancer. Lancet 1962 II b, 1235.

— — THOMAS, B. S.: The relation between the urinary 17-hydroxycorticosteroids and the 11-deoxy-17-oxosteroids and the fate of patients after mastectomy. Lancet 1964 I, 945.

DESHPANDE, N., BULBROOK, R. D.: A method for the simultaneous determination of 17-oxosteroids and 17-hydroxycorticosteroids in human plasma. J. Endocr. 28, 289 (1964).

— HAYWARD, J. L., BULBROOK, R. D.: Plasma 17-hydroxycorticosteroids and 17-oxosteroids in patients with breast cancer and in normal women. J. Endocr. 32, 167 (1965).

GALLAGHER, T. F., HELLMAN, L., BRADLOW, H. L., ZUMOFF, B., FUKUSHIMA, D. K.: The effect of thyroid hormones on the metabolism of steroids. Ann. N. Y. Acad. Sci. 86, 605 (1960).

GUTIERREZ, R. M., WILLIAMS, R. J.: Excretion of ketosteroids and proneness to breast cancer. Biochemistry 59, 938 (1968).

HAYWARD, J. L.: Steroid excretion in early breast cancer. Brit. J. Surg. 51, 224 (1964).

— The presymptomatic diagnosis of breast cancer. Proc. roy. Soc. Med. 59, 1204 (1966).

JURET, P., HAYEM, M., FLAISLER, A.: A propos de 150 implantations d'yttrium radio-actif intrahypophysaires dans le traitement du cancer du sein à un stade avancé. J. Chir. (Paris) 87, 409 (1964).

KUMAOKA, S., SAKAUCHI, N., ABE, O., KUSAMA, M., TAKATANI, O.: Urinary 17-ketosteroid excretion of women with advanced breast cancer. J. clin. Endocr. 28, 666 (1968).

MARMORSTON, J., CROWLEY, L. G., MYERS, S. M., STERN, E., HOPKINS, C. E.: Urinary excretion of neutral 17-ketosteroids and pregnanediol by patients with breast cancer and benign breast disease. Amer. J. Obstet. Gynec. 92, 447 (1965).

MILLER, H., DURANT, J. A.: The value of urine steroid hormone assays in breast cancer. Clin. Biochem. 1, 286 (1968).

MOOR, P., DE HENDRIKS, A., STEENO, O.: Ideopathic lowering of the cortisol binding capacity of human plasma transcortin. Ann. endocr. (Paris) 26, 488 (1965).

SCHWEPPE, J. S., JUNGMAN, R. A., LEWIN, I.: Urine steroid excretion in postmenopausal cancer of the breast. Cancer 20, 155 (1967).

SHAPIRO, S., STRAX, P., VENET, L.: Periodic breast cancer screening. Arch. environm. Hlth 15, 547 (1967).

SNEDDON, A., STEEL, J. M., STRONG, J. A.: Effect of thyroid function and of obesity on discriminant function for mammary carcinoma. Lancet 1968 II, 892.

WAARD, F. DE, BAANDERS-VAN HALEWIJN, E. A., HUIZINGA, J.: The bimodal age distribution of patients with mammary carcinoma. Cancer 17, 141 (1964).

WADE, A. P., DAVIS, J. C., TWEEDIE, M. C. K., CLARKE, C. A., HAGGART, B.: The discriminant function in early carcinoma of the breast. Lancet 1969 I, 853.

WANG, D. Y., HAYWARD, J. L., BULBROOK, R. D.: Testosteron levels in the plasma of normal women and patients with benign breast disease or with breast cancer. Europ. J. Cancer 2, 373 (1966).

Chapter 10

Pituitary and Thyroid Hormones

In man, direct attempts to correlate measurements of pituitary function with the development of breast tumours or with the clinical course of the disease have been unsuccessful. To some extent this may have been due to lack of accurate methods for measuring the amounts of pituitary hormones in plasma and urine—for instance there is still no way of estimating prolactin activity separate from that of growth hormone—but even allowing for this, and on those occasions when reasonably accurate methods of assay have been used, very few associations have been demonstrated between pituitary function and tumour growth or response to therapy.

1. Gonadotrophins

The measurement of urinary gonadotrophins involves many of the difficulties associated with the measurement of oestrogens; there is variation with age and also variation through the menstrual cycle. A further complication is that the measurements of the urinary excretion of gonadotrophin by breast cancer patients have been done using a bioassay technique. It now seems that this method is extremely insensitive and much of the work to date may have to be discounted. Probably use of the newer radio-immunoassays will clarify the situation.

LORAINE (1958) measured gonadotrophin excretion in forty-seven postmenopausal women with breast cancer before they were treated with stilboestrol. The urine specimens were collected over eight days and the mean excretion values were calculated from determinations on four 48-hour pools. Such was the variability that in some patients there was a two-fold difference in the gonadotrophin levels between samples. Similar assays were carried out on a control group of thirty-seven women suffering from diseases other than cancer. LORAINE noted that the patients who failed to respond to stilboestrol therapy had a significantly higher mean gonadotrophin excretion than the patients who obtained a remission. On the other hand, values in the remission group and the controls were almost identical. Thus the patients who were hormone unresponsive had abnormally high levels of urinary gonadotrophin whereas the levels of those who responded were well within the normal range. This is a similar phenomenon to that reported by BULBROOK et al. (1962) when investigating androgen excretion; they found that in patients with advanced breast cancer, normal excretion of 17-OHCS and aetiocholanolone only occurred in those who subsequently responded to adrenalectomy and hypophysectomy; abnormal levels were associated with subsequent failure to respond.

BOYLAND et al. (1958) measured the gonadotrophin excretion in thirty women with breast cancer before and after pituitary destruction by implantation of 198 Au or 90 Yttrium. They also found that the pre-treatment levels in the unresponsive patients tended to be high, although the numbers were very small.

On the other hand, HAYWARD, BULBROOK and GREENWOOD (1961) estimated the urinary gonadotrophins in 41 patients with advanced breast cancer who were awaiting adrenalectomy or hypophysectomy. Although the difference between the levels in the responsive and unresponsive patients was not significant, they found that the high levels tended to be in those who subsequently responded to ablation. These high levels were not found in patients who had had androgen or oestrogen therapy during the previous eight weeks.

Not all measurements of gonadotrophins in patients with breast cancer have shown a similar correlation with the subsequent response to endocrine therapy. BECK and his colleagues (1966) estimated the urinary gonadotrophins before and after hypophysectomy. They were able to demonstrate the expected drop in levels following removal of the pituitary gland but could find no marked correlation between the pre-operative values and response. They found that there was a considerable overlap between the pre-operative levels in the responsive and unresponsive patients but that the tendency was for the responsive to have high levels and the unresponsive to have low levels—the opposite to that noted by BOYLAND et al. (1958) but similar to the findings of HAYWARD et al. (1961). Similarly, MARTIN (1964) carried out 166 assays of urinary gonadotrophins in postmenopausal women with carcinoma of the breast. He reported that there was a significantly lower excretion of gonadotrophins in women with advanced breast cancer who were unresponsive to hormone therapy and in "poor" clinical condition. He also measured the urinary gonadotrophins in women after mastectomy who had not had a recurrence of the disease and compared these with the levels in women who had developed metastases. He showed that, the levels were significantly lower in those with metastases than in those without. However, there are several features in MARTIN's study that make it unsatisfactory. Firstly, his assays were carried out on two 24-hour specimens, sometimes collected twelve months apart; secondly, his "hormone therapy" included almost every treatment known to affect the advanced disease—androgens, oestrogens, corticosteroids, adrenalectomy and hypophysectomy; thirdly, his assessment of response was far from precise and included patients who had had only subjective improvement.

The evidence on alterations in gonadotrophin excretion in breast cancer patients and on the correlation of measurements with response to hormone therapy is conflicting. More study is needed using precise assay techniques and groups of patients that are as homogeneous as possible.

2. Growth Hormone and Prolactin

The story of the measurement of the pituitary protein hormones is a far from happy one. An accurate method for the estimation by a radio-immunoassay technique (HUNTER and GREENWOOD, 1964) of human growth hormone in plasma has only recently become available and any bio-assays previously carried out must be considered suspect.

Similarly the measurement of human prolactin has been restricted by difficulties in distinguishing prolactin activity from that of growth hormone. Purified growth

hormone has been found always to have considerable prolactin activity and there
have been doubts whether in man the two hormones are separate entities (see for
instance CHADWICK, FOLLEY and GEMZELL, 1961; TASHJIAN, LEVINE and WILHELMI,
1965). BOOT (1969) reviewed the literature and concluded that, although human
growth hormone may have some prolactin like activity, there is firm evidence of
the existence of two distinct hormones which by *in vitro* studies can be shown to
behave independently.

Interest in the effect of pituitary hormones on the growth of human breast cancer followed the demonstration of the part they played in the development of the
normal breast. LYONS (1943, 1958) and his collaborators provided evidence that in
castrated hypophysectomised weanling male rats both prolactin and growth hormone,
with the ovarian hormones, were necessary for the development of the mammary
gland. But the precise combinations of hormones responsible for ductal growth,
acinar development and the changes in pregnancy and lactation are extremely complex and not precisely understood in animals or man. Comprehensive reviews of the
literature have been given by COWIE and FOLLEY (1955) and LYONS (1958).

In humans, SCOWEN and HADFIELD (1955) attempted to measure the mammotrophic activity of female urine, assuming that any such activity might result in
part from the presence of protein hormones derived from the pituitary. They injected an extract of premenopausal female urine into weanling male rats and observed a marked acceleration in the growth of the duct system of the breast. They
showed that the urine extract contained no oestrogenic activity and, because the
extract was prepared by a method identical with that used for gonadotrophin assay,
they suggested that the mammotrophic activity was probably hypophysial in origin.
Further experiments showed that the duct growth which followed injection of the
urine extracts was similar to that obtained from the administration of prolactin
(HADFIELD and STRETTON YOUNG, 1956 a and b). Subsequent investigations, using
hypophysectomised weanling male mice, strongly suggested that the mammotrophic
agent in female urine was prolactin (HADFIELD, 1956 and 1958).

It was hoped that the method could be developed as an assay of the "mammotrophic potency" of human urine which might be of value in predicting the likely
response to hypophysectomy of patients with breast cancer (HADFIELD, 1956). The
work was extended using samples of serum as well as urine, but there were considerable methodological problems. In particular, it was difficult to find a strain of
mice which was sensitive to the extracts and retained this sensitivity. FRASER et al.
(1961) confirmed that the activity in normal female urine and serum was the property of prolactin and of growth hormone but found that the variability of response
was immense. Further simplification of the technique did not affect the variability
and they concluded that the method was unsuitable for quantitative assays.

Nevertheless the response of human breast cancer to additive or ablative procedures cannot be explained solely on alterations of androgen and oestrogen production, and a proper understanding of the effects of prolactin activity in these patients
may be essential to our understanding of the behaviour of the disease.

There is evidence from animal work that further investigation may be fruitful.
PEARSON (1967) has shown in rats that DMBA induced mammary tumours, which
have regressed following adrenalectomy or hypophysectomy, can be reactivated by
sheep prolactin. On the other hand, bovine growth hormone, oestrogen or pro-

gesterone, or a combination of these hormones fails to act on these tumours after the animal has been hypophysectomised. PEARSON hesitates to apply these data to man but suggests the need for further study of the part played by prolactin in human breast cancer. He has also administered human growth hormone for short periods to a few patients who had undergone surgical hypophysectomy for breast cancer. Whether the hormone was given with or without oestrogen, there was no reactivation of tumour growth.

Using hypophysial isografts, BOOT (1969) showed that excessive stimulation by prolactin and progesterone in the presence of normal oestrogens, growth hormone, and corticosteroids causes mammary tumours in mice. He confirmed this carcinogenic activity by inducing breast tumours in mice following the injection of ovine prolactin over a long period.

Providing prolactin exists as a separate hormone in the human, an accurate assay technique should be attainable. Probably a radio-immunoassay will eventually be evolved, similar to that now available for the measurement of growth hormone.

The availability of a radio-immunological method for the assay of human growth hormone in plasma has allowed precise measurements to be made in patients with breast cancer. But there are still many variables that have to be taken into account. GREENWOOD and LANDON (1966) have described some of the factors which affect plasma growth hormone levels. So many of these are functions of normal physiology, e. g. stress, exercise, fasting, insulin, etc., that measurements of plasma growth hormone can only be meaningful in strictly controlled conditions.

A standard stimulus has provided the most appropriate conditions for study, and GREENWOOD and his colleagues (1967, 1968) have used the growth hormone response to insulin-induced hypoglycaemia. In ten patients with early breast cancer, they measured the rise in plasma growth hormone and plasma cortisol levels both before and after radical mastectomy (the rise in plasma cortisol is in response to the increased secretion of ACTH, also resulting from the insulin load). Although the resting levels of growth hormone and cortisol were high, following a stimulus of 0.1 units of insulin per kilogramme body weight the rise in the levels of both hormones was normal.

On the other hand, PEARSON and his coworkers (1967, 1968) have described a paradoxical rise in serum growth hormone levels in nine out of twenty-three patients with advanced mammary cancer undergoing glucose tolerance tests. In normal subjects, serum growth hormone falls to immeasurable levels after a glucose load. PEARSON thought the paradoxical rise was probably due to an abnormal regulation of growth hormone secretion but noted that it did not appear to correlate with the subsequent response of the patients to endocrine ablation. GREENWOOD (1968) believes that these abnormalities in carbohydrate metabolism found in breast cancer patients may be a feature of the age of the patients.

Thyroid

The concept that thyroid function and the development of breast cancer could be interrelated is not new, nor is the idea that thyroid administration could have a beneficial effect on the progress of the established disease. BEATSON (1896), in his original paper on the use of oophorectomy in breast cancer, described how he gave his patients thyroid extract as adjunctive therapy. But the results from thyroid therapy were not promising and from BEATSON's day until the early 1950's, interest in the subject was sporadic. Most physicians felt that the activity of the thyroid gland played only a minor supportive role in the development and treatment of breast cancer and that little worthwhile would result from further investigation.

In the last fifteen years, interest has re-awakened and reports have now appeared linking the thyroid gland and breast cancer in respect of aetiology, development and treatment. The evidence of an association is still incomplete but sufficient data are now available for an assessment to be attempted.

1. Thyroid Disease and the Incidence of Breast Cancer

Most reports have inferred a positive correlation between the incidence of breast cancer and a history of thyroid disease or hypothyroidism. In 1952, REPERT investigated the incidence of thyroid disease in 305 patients with breast cancer and found the rate to be ten times that expected. LOESER (1954) believed that hypothyroid patients had a higher incidence of breast cancer than normal women. He also claimed that the incidence of recurrence of breast cancer after mastectomy was reduced in patients treated with thyroid extract. Throughout his life, LOESER continued to champion the cause of thyroid treatment in breast cancer but little attention was paid to his claims. ELLERKER (1956) reported on the breast pathology of 100 women who had previously undergone thyroidectomy and found a 6 per cent incidence of breast cancer. He also reviewed the history of 107 women with breast cancer and found a 7.6 per cent incidence of goitre. He concluded that thyroid disease and breast cancer were associated and that this association was more pronounced than could be expected by chance. SOMMERS (1955) carried out postmortem examinations of the endocrine glands and target organs in 707 women with breast cancer and 248 controls. He noticed a greater number of patients in the cancer group with hyperplastic changes in the ovaries, endometrium, uninvolved breast and in the pituitary and adrenal cortex. He also noted that only 14 per cent of the breast cancer patients had normal thyroid glands, compared with 65 per cent of the controls. Converse but supportive evidence was supplied by WYNDER et al. (1960) in their epidemiological study of breast cancer. They reported that a history of hyperthyroidism was less common in their patients with breast cancer than in their control group.

Further supportive evidence was given by BOGARDUS and FINLEY (1961). In their study of 79 patients with breast cancer, they found that forty-two patients had some thyroid abnormality—usually a goitre. None of their patients was hyperthyroid. BACKWINKEL and JACKSON (1964) also investigated their breast cancer patients for evidence of hypothyroidism. They found that 52 out of 280 patients with breast cancer or 18.5 per cent were hypothyroid. But they remarked that this high incidence of thyroid deficiency did not prove a causal relationship with breast cancer as it reflected the overall incidence of goitre within the particular age group studied and within that geographical region. They further commented that although the incidence of goitre had declined sharply in the United States of America since 1924, the death rate from breast cancer was unaltered. HUMPHREY and SWERDLOW

(1964) reviewed 196 patients who had been followed up for twelve years after having a thyroidectomy for hyperthyroidism or nontoxic goitre. During this period, no patient developed a carcinoma of the breast. Conversely, they found that two per cent of 369 patients, operated on for carcinoma of the breast had a history of thyroid disease.

CHALSTREY and BENJAMIN (1966) investigated the incidence of breast cancer amongst female patients who had been treated for thyroid cancer. Of 92 patients who had been treated during the twenty year period 1945—1964, eight of them (8.7 per cent) also had carcinoma of the breast. They then compared their results with the incidence of breast cancer shown in the National Cancer Register. They found that the national incidence of breast cancer in women aged over thirty five was 0.1 per cent, which was far below their figure of 8.7 per cent for the thyroid cancer patients. However, they failed to take into account that the national incidence was calculated from the number of cases of breast cancer occurring during one year, whilst the incidence in their cases had been accumulated over 27 years. In effect, no comparison can be made without an equivalent time scale of observation. The usual expected incidence of breast cancer is about 4 to 4.5 per cent in the total female population, so CHALSTREY and BENJAMIN's figure of 8.7 per cent is certainly high. When all their thyroid cancer patients have died, a more accurate comparison can be made but it appears that the observed incidence of breast cancer in their patients will be something over twice the expected incidence.

These reports give presumptive evidence of an association between thyroid disease and the incidence of breast cancer. The most constant finding is that breast cancer occurs more commonly in hypothyroid patients and possibly less commonly in hyperthyroid patients. The numbers involved are not large and, although of epidemiological interest, the association seems to have little practical importance. It seems likely that if an endocrine factor can be demonstrated in the aetiology of breast cancer, then hypothyroidism may occasionally play an initiating role in the hormone changes that are required to stimulate neoplasia.

2. Thyroid Factors in the Established Disease

Many workers have attempted to detect abnormalities in thyroid function in patients with established breast cancer. The changes in thyroid activity which may accompany progressive dissemination of the disease have also been investigated. EDELSTYN et al. (1958) found that patients with localised breast cancer were euthyroid, but patients with metastatic disease had diminished thyroid function. Similarly, CARTER et al. (1960) could detect no difference between the serum protein bound iodine levels in postmenopausal normal women and in patients who had been successfully treated for early breast cancer. When they investigated patients with disseminated disease, the serum protein bound iodine levels were significantly higher.

STOLL (1965) studied ^{131}I uptake in patients with breast cancer, patients "cured" of breast cancer and normal women, but could find no evidence of altered thyroid function. In a small group of patients with large necrotic tumours, he was able to demonstrate an extremely low ^{131}I uptake and suggested that if a high percentage of such patients were in a study group, this could account for the reports of low thyroid function in breast cancer. Other similar investigations by REEVE et al. (1961)

and CAPELLI and MARGOTTINI (1964) failed to show any change in thyroid function in patients with breast cancer but a conflicting report comes from BIGNAZZI and VERONESE (1965). They studied forty seven patients with operable breast cancer and compared them with forty one normal controls. Following administration of ^{131}I, thyroid function was measured by estimating the uptake of radioactive iodine by the thyroid and by determining the quantity of protein bound radioactive iodine in the plasma. The breast cancer patients were found to have a significantly higher uptake than the controls both at three and twenty four hours after administration of the [131]I. These workers were unable to demonstrate any abnormality of thyroid activity in a few patients with osseous metastases.

A somewhat different approach to the problem has been to try to detect an association between thyroid function and prognosis in patients with breast cancer. HUMPHREY and SWERDLOW (1964) investigated the survival and incidence of recurrence in breast cancer patients having a history of thyroid disease, and compared them with a similar group having no history of thyroid disease. There was a lower incidence of local recurrence in the group with a thyroid history than in the controls (6.8 per cent, compared with 13.8 per cent). Also the five year survival rate was 71 per cent in patients who had had a thyroidectomy for nontoxic goitre, compared with 47.4 per cent for those without thyroid disease. BACKWINKEL and JACKSON (1964) also observed a longer survival time in patients dying from breast cancer who were hypothyroid than those who were euthyroid (35 months, compared with 30 months). SICHER and WATERHOUSE (1967) also tried to assess the influence of thyroid activity on prognosis in breast cancer. They used the uptake of ^{131}I and the level of serum protein bound iodine as measures of thyroid activity. The patients were followed up for five years and their survival was related to the initial measurements. No correlation was detected but SICHER and WATERHOUSE inclined to attribute this to the possible use of inappropriate methods for measuring thyroid activity. They proposed to attempt a further assessment of the potential of the thyroid gland by including measurements of the response to exogenous stimulation.

These many reports seem to have contributed little to our understanding of the problem. There is no conclusive evidence on the thyroid status of patients with breast cancer, either in the early or late stages—although there is some suggestion that the latter patients may tend to be hypothyroid. Similarly, the data on thyroid function and prognosis seem inconclusive. There is some evidence that a correlation may exist but it is difficult to demonstrate. Possibly, further prospective trials, as suggested by SICHER and WATERHOUSE, may throw further light on the problem.

3. Thyroid as Treatment

Thyroid hormone has had rather a chequered career as a treatment for breast cancer. It has been prescribed mostly in the management of the advanced disease, although LOESER (1954) used it as a prophylactic measure after mastectomy. On many occasions, partly to combat the possible development of hypothyroidism, thyroid extract or triodothyronine has been used in combination with prednisone. Hence it has been difficult to distinguish between the remissions due to the thyroid and those due to the prednisone (see for instance LEMON, 1957; GARDNER et al., 1962). The success rate from combined thyroid and prednisone therapy is not high—

GARDNER et al. (1962) reported 24 per cent with an average duration of six months, but this response could be completely accounted for by the effect of the steroid alone. Evidence suggesting that thyroid has little value as a treatment for breast cancer comes from EMERY and TROTTER (1963). They undertook a controlled clinical trial in which patients with advanced breast cancer were randomly selected for treatment with triodothyronine. They concluded from their results that the compound had no therapeutic effect in these circumstances.

4. Thyroid Effects on Endocrine Metabolism

There is an extremely complex interrelation between the action of different hormones. Variation in the secretion or metabolism of one hormone can have a profound effect on the secretion or metabolism of another. Thus any effect that hypo or hyperthyroidism may have on the aetiology and development of breast cancer may be mediated through reactions involving other hormones. For instance, it is known that the level of thyroid hormone affects the metabolic transformation of certain steroid hormones. Testosterone and dehydroepiandrosterone are largely converted to metabolites of the androstane series in conditions where the levels of thyroid hormone are elevated (HELLMAN et al., 1959). Hyperthyroid patients excrete increased amounts of the 17-OHCS whereas in hypothyroid patients the 17-OHCS excretion is less than normal. Also hypothyroid patients excrete subnormal amounts of aetiocholanolone and androsterone (SNEDDON et al., 1968). Thyroid hormone has been shown to influence the metabolism of administeroid oestradiol—16-C14. In conditions where the levels of thyroid hormone are elevated, there is a decrease in the fraction converted to oestriol and an increase in the fraction converted to to 2-methoxyoestrone (FISHMAN et al., 1962). Almost certainly, the metabolism of other hormones derived from the ovary or adrenal is altered in conditions of hypo or hyperthyroidism. Conversely, the secretion of thyroid hormone is in its turn affected by alterations in adrenal and ovarian secretion. The complexity of the interrelationship between the thyroid and the adrenal cortex has been summarised by GOLDENBERG et al. (1966):

"... The consensus of opinion leads inexorably to the following simplifications:

a) administration of adrenocortical steroids causes suppression of thyroid function.

b) removal of adrenocortical influences allows thyroid activity to increase;

c) increase of thyroid hormone is followed by increased adrenocortical effects;

d) decreased thyroid function is followed by decreased adrenocortical function."

Thus, there appear to be both antagonistic and synergistic effects resulting from initial alterations in functional levels of thyroid or adrenal hormones.

Attempts at an analysis of the metabolic effects that may occur in hypothyroidism and their possible relationship with the development of breast cancer have been made only at the most superficial level. The precise alterations in adrenal and ovarian metabolism, which may be associated with the development of breast cancer and also have their effect on thyroid secretion, have proved extremely complex. It is impossible to know at the moment which function of the endocrine glands initiates the minor alterations of thyroid function which are observed in some patients with breast cancer.

Summary and Conclusions

1. The findings on the levels of urinary gonadotrophins in patients with breast cancer and on the correlation of these levels with response to treatment are conflicting. This may result from the use of insensitive methods of assay.

2. Prolactin can be carcinogenic in mice but there is no evidence of a similar effect in man. As yet, there is no method of measuring prolactin activity in man separate from that of growth hormone.

3. Using radio-immunoassay techniques, no consistent abnormality of growth hormone secretion has been detected in breast cancer patients.

4. There is some evidence that breast cancer occurs more commonly in patients with a history of hypothyroidism and less commonly in those with a history of hyperthyroidism.

5. There is no conclusive evidence of abnormal thyroid function in patients with early or advanced breast cancer. No definite correlation has been demonstrated between thyroid function and prognosis.

6. The treatment of breast cancer with thyroid hormones is ineffective.

7. The mechanism of the alterations in thyroid metabolism which precede the onset of breast cancer is unknown.

References

BACKWINKEL, K., JACKSON, A. S.: Some features of breast cancer and thyroid deficiency. Report of 280 cases. Cancer 17, 1174 (1964).

BEATSON, G. T.: On the treatment of inoperable cases of carcinoma of the mamma; suggestions for a new method of treatment with illustrative cases. Lancet 1896 II, 104, 162.

BECK, J. C., BLAIR, A. J., GRIFFITHS, M. M., ROSENFELD, M. W., McGARRY, E. E.: In search of hormonal factors as an aid in predicting the outcome of breast carcinoma. In: Proceedings of the Sixth Canadian Cancer Conference. Ed.: R. W. BEGG. Oxford: Pergamon Press 1966, p. 3.

BIGNAZZI, D. B., VERONESI, U.: Thyroid function in patients with cancer of the breast. Surg. Gynec. Obstet. 20, 1132 (1965).

BOGARDUS, G. M., FINLEY, J. W.: Breast cancer and thyroid disease. Surgery 49, 461 (1961).

BOOT, L. M.: Induction by prolactin of mammary tumours in mice. Academisch Proefschrift, Noord-Hollandse. Amsterdam 1969.

BOYLAND, E., GODSMARK, B., GREENING, W. P., RIGBY-JONES, P., STEVENSON, J. J., ABUL-FADL, M. A. M.: The effect of irradiation of the pituitary on gonadotrophin excretion in women with advanced mammary cancer. In: Endocrine Aspects of Breast Cancer. Ed.: A. P. CURRIE. Edinburgh-London: Livingstone 1958, p. 170.

BULBROOK, R. D., HAYWARD, J. L., SPICER, C. C., THOMAS, B. S.: A comparison between the urinary steroid excretion of normal women and women with advanced breast cancer. Lancet 1962 II, 1235.

CAPELLI, L., MARGOTTINI, M.: Thyroid function in cancer patients. Acta. Un. int. Cancr. 20, 1493 (1964).

CARTER, A. C., FELDMAN, E. B., SCHWARTZ, H. L.: Levels of serum protein-bound iodine in patients with metastatic carcinoma of the breast. J. clin. Endocr. 20, 477 (1960).

CHADWICK, A., FOLLEY, S. J., GEMZELL, C. A.: Lactogenic activity of human pituitary growth hormone. Lancet 1961 II, 241.

CHALSTREY, L. J., BENJAMIN, B.: High incidence of breast cancer in thyroid cancer patients. Brit. J. Cancer 20, 670 (1966).

COWIE, A. T., FOLLEY, J. S.: In: The Hormones, Vol. 3. Eds.: G. PINGUS and K. V. THIMANN. New York: Academic Press 1955, p. 309.

EDELSTYN, G. A., LYONS, A. R., WELBOURN, R. B.: Thyroid function in patients with mammary cancer. Lancet 1958 I, 670.

ELLERKER, A. G.: Thyroid disorders in breast cancer, a causal connection? Med. Press 235, 280 (1956).

EMERY, E. W., TROTTER, W. R.: Triiodothyronine in advanced breast cancer. Lancet 1963 I, 358.

FISHMAN, J., HELLMAN, L., ZUMOFF, B., GALLAGHER, T. F.: Influence of thyroid hormone on oestrogen metabolism in man. J. clin. Endocr. 22, 389 (1962).

FRASER, L. E., SPICER, C. C., WILLIAMS, P. C., YOUNG, STRETTON: Detection and attempted assay of mammotrophic activity in women's blood and urine. Brit. J. Cancer 15, 243 (1961).

GARDNER, B., THOMAS, A. N., GORDAN, G. S.: Antitumor efficacy of prednisone and liothyronine in advanced breast cancer. Cancer 15, 334 (1962).

GOLDENBERG, I. S., BLODINGER, P. H., GRUMMON, R. A.: Some observations on thyroid-adrenocortical interrelationships. Surgery 59, 522 (1966).

GREENWOOD, F. C.: Biological problems regarding hormonal surgery. In: Major Endocrine Surgery for the Treatment of Cancer of the Breast in Advanced Stages. Eds.: M. DARGENT and CL. ROMIEU. Lyon: Simep Editions 1967, p. 199.

— Personal communication (1968).

— JAMES, V. H. T., MEGGITT, B. F., MILLER, J. D., TAYLOR, P. H.: Pituitary function in breast cancer. In: Prognostic Factors in Breast Cancer. Eds.: A. P. M. FORREST and P. B. KUNKLER. Edinburgh-London: Livingstone 1968, p. 409.

— LANDON, J.: Assessment of hypothalamic pituitary function in endocrine disease. J. clin. Path. 19, 284 (1966).

HADFIELD, G.: Mammotrophic potency in human urine. In: Endocrine aspects of breast cancer. Ed.: A. R. CURRIE. Edinburgh-London: Livingstone 1958, p. 174.

— Recent research in physiology of breast applied to mammary cancer. Brit. Med. J. 1, 1507 (1956).

— YOUNG, STRETTON: The mammotrophic potency of human urine. Brit. J. Cancer 10, 145 (1956 a).

— — The mammotrophic potency of the urine of normal premenopausal women. Brit. J. Cancer 10, 325 (1956 b).

HAYWARD, J. L., BULBROOK, R. D., GREENWOOD, F. C.: Hormone assays and prognosis in breast cancer. Mem. Soc. Endocr. 10, 144 (1961).

HELLMAN, L., BRADLOW, H. L., ZUMOFF, B., FUKUSHIMA, D. K., GALLAGHER, T. F.: Thyroid-androgen interrelations and the hypercholesteremic effect of androsterone. J. clin. Endocr. 19, 936 (1959).

HUMPHREY, L. J., SWERDLOW, M.: The relationship of breast disease to thyroid disease. Cancer 17, 1170 (1964).

HUNTER, W. M., GREENWOOD, F. C.: A radio-immunoelectrophoretic assay for human growth hormone. Biochem. J. 91, 43 (1964).

LEMON, H. M.: Cortisone-thyroid therapy of metastatic mammary cancer. Ann. int. Med. 46, 457 (1957).

LOESER, A. A.: A new therapy for prevention of postoperative recurrence in genital and breast cancer; 6 years study of prophylactic thyroid treatment. Brit. med. J. 1954 II, 1380.

LORAINE, J. A.: The estimation of anterior pituitary hormones in patients with mammary carcinoma. In: Endocrine Aspects of Breast Cancer. Ed.: A. P. CURRIE. Edinburgh-London: Livingstone 1958, p. 158.

LYONS, W. R.: Hormonal synergism in mammary growth. Proc. roy. Soc. B 149, 303 (1958).

— Lobulo-alveolar mammary growth induced in hypophysectomised rats by injection of ovarian and hypophysical hormones. Essays in Biol. 315 (1943).

MARTIN, F. I. R.: Urinary gonadotrophins in post-menopausal women with breast cancer. Brit. med. J. 1964 II, 351.

PEARSON, O. H.: Biological problems regarding hormonal surgery. In: Major Endocrine Surgery for the Treatment of Cancer of the Breast in Advanced Stages. Eds.: M. DARGENT and CL. ROMIEU. Lyon: Simep Editions 1967, p. 215.

— LLERENA, O., SAMAAN, N., GONZALEZ, D.: Serum growth hormone and insulin levels in patients with breast cancer. In: Prognostic Factors in Breast Cancer. Eds.: A. P. M. FORREST and P. B. KUNKLER. Edinburgh-London: Livingstone 1968, p. 421.

REEVE, T. S., RUNDLE, F. F., HAYLES, I. B., MYHILL, J., CROYDON, M.: Thyroid function in the presence of breast cancer. Lancet 1961 I, 632.

REPERT, R. W.: Breast carcinoma study: relation to thyroid disease and diabetes. J. Mich. med. Soc. 51, 1315 (1952).

SCOWEN, E. F., HADFIELD, G.: Mammotrophic activity of extracts of human urine. Cancer 8, 890 (1955).

SICHER, K., WATERHOUSE, J. A. H.: Thyroid function in relation to prognosis in mammary cancer. Brit. J. Cancer 21, 512 (1967).

SNEDDON, A., STEEL, J. M., STRONG, J. A.: Effect of thyroid function and of obesity on discriminant function for mammary carcinoma. Lancet 1968 II, 892.

SOMMERS, S. C.: Endocrine abnormalities in women with breast cancer. Lab. Invest. (Philadelphia) 4, 160 (1955).

STOLL, B. A.: Breast Cancer and Hypothyroidism. Cancer 18, 1431 (1965).

TASHJIAN, A. H., LEVINE, L., WILHELMI, A. E.: Immunochemical studies with antisera to fractions of human growth hormone which are high or low in pigeon crop gland-stimulating activity. Endocrinology 77, 1023 (1965).

WYNDER, E. L., BROSS, I. J., HIRAYAMA, T.: A study of the epidemiology of cancer of the breast. Cancer 13, 559 (1960).

Chapter 11

The Present and the Future

There is now evidence that the sex linkage in breast cancer can be accounted for by differences in the hormonal environment between men and women. The incidence in men can be increased probably to a rate similar to that in the female by the administration of oestrogens or by feminising conditions; also, there is evidence that men with breast cancer metabolise oestrogen abnormally.

The prescription of oestrogens to women does not have the same effect; moreover, there is only circumstantial evidence that endogenous hyperoestrogenism may be associated with a high incidence of breast cancer—and this only in postmenopausal women—and reports of alterations of oestrogen excretion in women with the established disease have been conflicting. On the other hand, there are now observations showing that many women with breast cancer have abnormalities in androgen and corticoid excretion. One investigation has indicated that these abnormalities may precede the onset of the disease.

Thus, although there is no direct evidence that androgens, oestrogens or indeed any known hormones are carcinogenic in men or women, certain abnormalities in the hormonal milieu, probably acting with other unknown agents, may condition breast tissue to neoplasia. These abnormalities are highly complex and may take different forms; that is to say, in certain circumstances, many different hormonal states may engender similar neoplastic changes. Providing the hormonal environment is favourable for neoplasia, local factors are likely to determine when the cancer appears and its siting within the breast.

Once neoplastic changes have occurred within the breast, these changes seem to be irreversible, or at least irreversable with our present methods of treatment. By altering the hormonal milieu from a favourable to an unfavourable one, the growth of the breast cancer can be halted and tumour tissue can even be destroyed, but inevitably the cancer adapts itself to this change and sooner or later will grow in the altered environment. Further environmental changes may again cause the neoplastic growth to stop; on occasions, even a reversion to the original hormonal environment will cause a remission.

Information on the environment in which these responsive tumours grow can now be obtained from blood or urinary hormone assays, and the results of these assays are of some value in predicting the response to endocrine treatment.

Although an oversimplification, these are the bones of our knowledge at the moment. What, then, are likely to be the developments in the immediate future?

It is difficult to see many advances being made in the hormonal treatment of breast cancer. Either a tumour is hormone responsive, and will react to environmental changes by regressing, or it is not. It is unlikely both that the unresponsive tumour can be made to respond and that the responsive tumour can be made to respond more profoundly. Of course, it is conceivable that tumours unresponsive to one hormone may respond to another, but this is unlikely to be a frequent occurrence. The most likely result of future research is that treatment will be placed on a more rational basis. More precise hormone assays, interpreted in the light of the clinical findings, will give a greater degree of prediction both of the likely response of the tumour and of the best agent for obtaining this response. Of greatest value in this field will be the selection of patients most likely to benefit from prophylactic therapy. Whether the therapy be hormone administration or endocrine ablation, accurate prediction will overcome the clinicians present dilemma in which he has to treat either all patients to help the few or no-one. This dilemma is complicated by the probability that the prescription of prophylactic therapy to some patients may cause the tumour to grow faster, a danger which is also present in the treatment of the advanced disease. Precise hormone assays giving detailed information on the favourable and unfavourable environments for each tumour should obviate much of this danger. Probably, not only the hormone environment but also the response of the tumour to this environment will have to be taken into account.

Results of investigations into the part played by hormones in the aetiology of breast cancer are encouraging. If it can be confirmed that a specific hormonal milieu conditions breast tissue to neoplastic change and if this milieu can be identified, we have gone a long way towards detecting women who are particularly susceptible. This might be possible whilst a woman is still young and long before the carcinoma has been initiated. It could result in the identification of a high risk group in which the incidence of breast cancer might be much greater than normal. Women in this group could be subjected to frequent examination so that a developing tumour could be detected whilst it was still localised. More sophisticated aids to clinical examination, such as mammography, thermography or xeroradiography, may be of help in screening this relatively small population.

An active attempt at prevention is another possibility which may follow the detection of the hormonal conditions most favourable for breast cancer. If it can be shown that abnormal hormone secretion or metabolism creates a favourable climate for the development of breast tumours, and if this state can be precisely identified, then it may be corrected. Possibly, the prescription of suitable hormones or the alteration of the activity of an enzyme system may effectively change the hormonal environment to one unfavourable to breast neoplasia.

On the debit side, there are two recurring problems which have profoundly affected the quality of the information obtained from research into the hormonal aspects of human breast cancer so far, and to which attention must be given in the future. First is the pattern of development of hormone assay methods. During the last twenty years, techniques of measurement of almost every hormone have changed, in some instances, many times. In most cases, this has necessitated the discarding of all previous recordings because they were either inaccurate, did not measure the substances they were designed to measure, or were insensitive to small quantitative changes. Inevitably, this has meant that a large amount of otherwise good work has had to be discarded. Most taxing of all is the fear that the results of many current investigations will also prove unacceptable as further refinements in techniques are introduced.

Possibly there is little that can be done about this. It would hardly be profitable to prevent improved methods of assay being introduced. Nevertheless, much of the rejected information represents many years labour by both scientists and clinicians, has cost a great deal of money—often donated—and, most important of all, resulted from the generous collaboration sometimes at great discomfort of many thousands of patients. It is the responsibility of all workers, whether in the laboratory or the hospital ward, critically to appraise the methods they use before undertaking an investigation.

The other problem, and one that has caused much unnecessary confusion ever since endocrine therapy was first introduced for breast cancer, is the lack of agreement on methods to assess the response of the patient. This has been mentioned before in these pages but, until proper steps are taken by the medical profession to bring order into the present chaos, it cannot be emphasised too often. It is quite ludicrous that, in these days when the controlled trial is really playing its part in the solution of many difficult clinical problems, work should be rendered invalid by the use of indefinite and often unacceptable criteria of clinical response. Possibly one of the international bodies such as the U.I.C.C. should accept the responsibility for getting agreement on this point.

Bearing in mind these strictures, the future otherwise appears encouraging. There are now forseeable goals which could be reached within the next two decades—early identification, accurate prediction and possibly prevention. If they are achieved, breast cancer could cease to be the commonest and most lethal tumour in women, and the treatment of those cases that occur should be more effective.

Type-setting, printing and binding: Konrad Triltsch, Graphischer Betrieb, 87 Würzburg, Germany

Monographs already Published

In Production

In Preparation